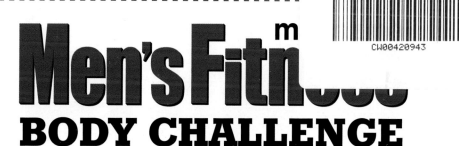

BODY CHALLENGE

By Pete Muir

Additional text **Lucy Miller, Ben Bradbury**
Photography **Tom Miles**
Design **Spike**
Model **Toby Rowland @ Nevs**
Subeditor **Juliet Giles**

For more information on *Men's Fitness* magazine, go to www.mensfitnessmagazine.co.uk.
To subscribe call 0844 844 0081.

Dennis Publishing
© Copyright Dennis Publishing Ltd. Licensed by Felden 2009

With thanks to

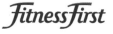

www.fitnessfirst.co.uk

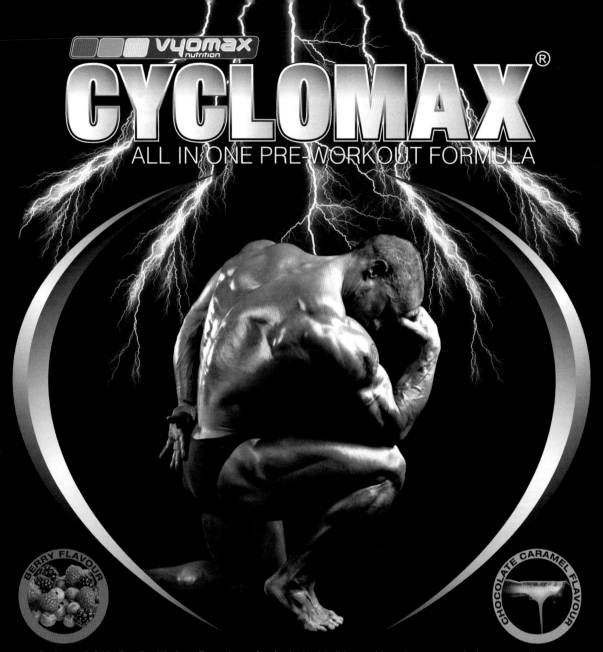
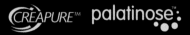

CONTENTS

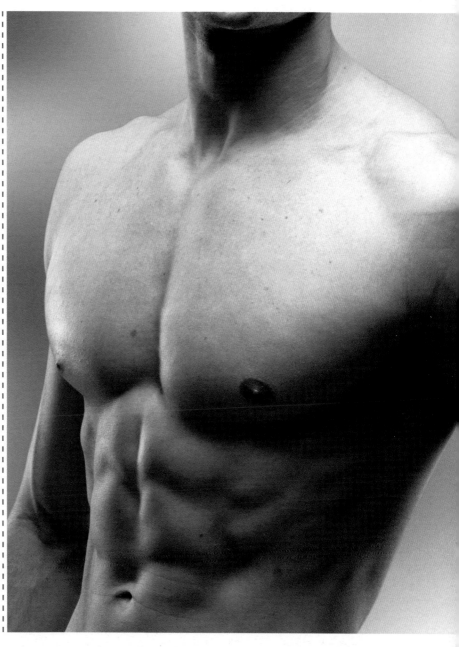

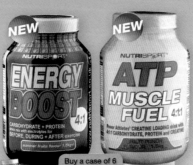
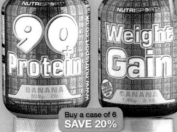
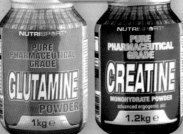
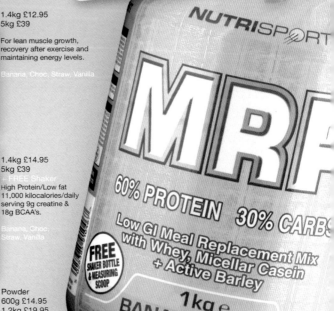
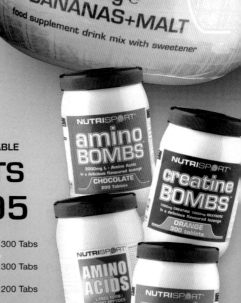

Take the challenge
Your 12-week journey to a new body starts here

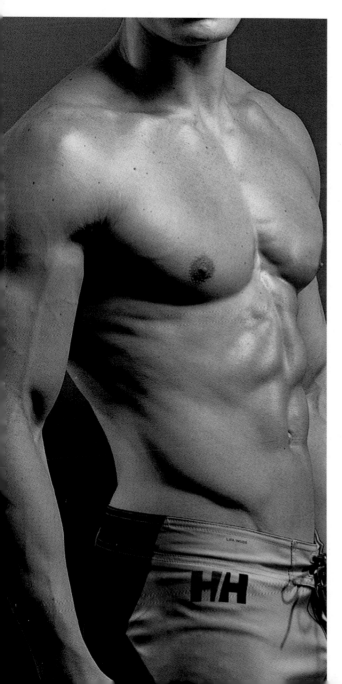

Lots of people would love to change their body shape. Not quite so many people know how to go about it properly. But that doesn't mean that an ideal body is beyond most people's reach.

In 12 weeks you can transform your body by stripping away fat and building new muscle to make yourself look leaner, firmer and more athletic. The best way to achieve this is through a combination of weight training, cardio and sensible eating – which is exactly what the *Men's Fitness Body Challenge* provides, with every exercise and every meal designed for you every day. What's more, this plan is suitable for everyone. The workouts are manageable for beginners, but will still help experienced gym-goers to see great results. And if you are short on time, each session shouldn't take more than 45 minutes, so you can fit it into your busy day. Start now and get the body you've always wanted, in less time than you thought possible.

Men's Fitness Body Challenge
WHAT YOU'LL GET

- ☑ Lose fat from all over your body

- ☑ Gain new muscle to look lean and hard

- ☑ Reveal your hidden six-pack

- ☑ Feel healthy and energised

- ☑ Train for no more than 45 minutes a day

- ☑ All workouts and meals planned for you

- ☑ Perfect for beginners or experienced gym-goers

- ☑ No fad diets or extreme training methods

- ☑ See great results in just 12 weeks

How it works

The 12-week Body Challenge plan explained

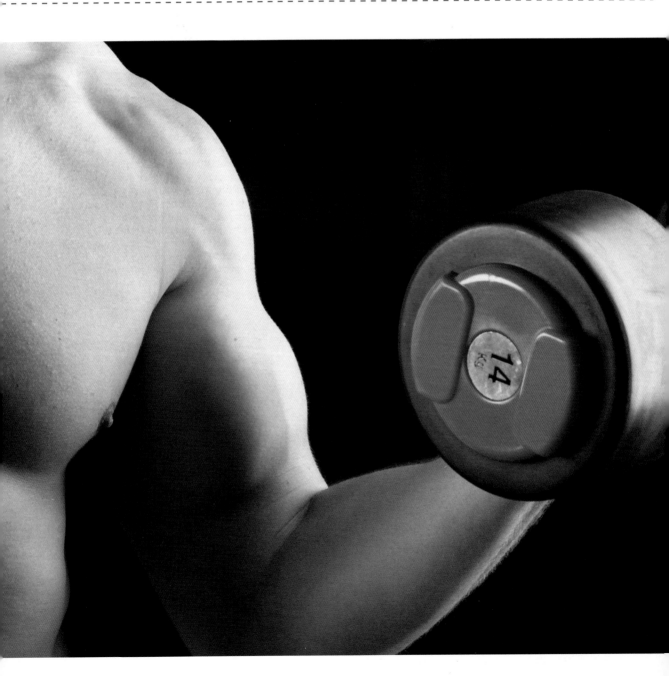

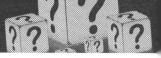

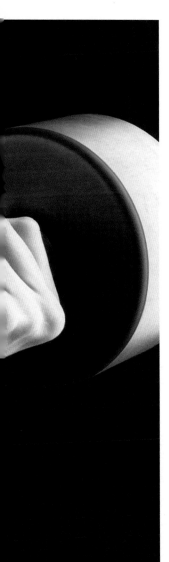

Transforming your body in a short space of time is perfectly achievable – but only if you give yourself every chance to succeed. In this book we'll give you all the training guides you need, plus nutrition plans and tips on getting the most from your workouts, but you need to commit to working hard and eating right. If you do that, we'll be with you every step of the way.

The workouts

A workout is a series of exercises, performed with a specific goal in mind. The type of exercises you do, the number of reps, the speed you perform them at, the weight you choose... all these things will affect the outcome your training. Fortunately, we have worked out all the variables for you. All you have to do is follow the plans to the letter to see great results in 12 weeks.

You'll do three weights-based workouts a week. This is enough to stress your muscles and stimulate them into more growth, while giving you sufficient time to rest and recover between workouts.

To start with, the workouts are designed to get your body used to training. You'll learn how to stabilise your own bodyweight and get your neuromuscular connections firing, so that your body adapts quickly and is ready for the harder work to come in later weeks.

At the start of each week you'll get an exercise plan for the week and a nutritional plan. Where it says 'Workout A', simply turn over the page and you'll find the workout laid out for you, with detailed explanations of how to perform each exercise. Each workout starts with a workout log, showing the order of exercises, the number of sets and reps, the tempo, rest and weight. Pay attention to all these figures when you do the workout, and if you're unsure what some of the figures mean, look at the terminology section on p10. You'll notice however, the final 'weight' column has been left blank, for you to fill in the values yourself once you have worked out what is the best resistance for you for each exercise.

Cardio sessions

As well as the weight training sessions, you'll also do two cardio sessions a week. Cardio (short for cardiovascular) training is designed to get your heart pumping in order to make it stronger and raise your overall fitness levels. As well as making you fitter and healthier, cardio training is a great way to burn off fat stores, and as long as you don't make your sessions too long, it won't affect your muscle growth.

The cardio sessions are outlined in the weekly training plans. You can choose which type of training you'd like to do – running, swimming, cycling, rowing or any other similar type of exercise – but running is the most efficient calorie burner, so we have focussed on that in most of the sessions.

Nutrition plans

Each week you will also get a comprehensive eating plan to go with your training plans. The calorie count is around 2,500-3,000 calories a day, which is enough to fuel your workouts and build new muscle. And because the meals are designed to provide the right balance of carbs, proteins and fats, you shouldn't put on any unwanted weight around your middle.

If you struggle to stick with the meal plans, either because you can't find the ingredients or your lifestyle makes following the plans awkward, we have also provided a selection of meals and snacks that you can use to build your own nutrition plans. See p20 for more details.

Rest days

Two days a week are designated as rest days. On these days you really should rest – take it easy, put your feet up, get plenty of sleep. It's important that you don't try to speed up your results by training on these days, because your body needs time to recover from the workouts in order to adapt and grow stronger. If you don't rest you'll find that your muscles don't grow, and you could suffer from over-training and become susceptible to illness.

Gym lingo

A quick guide to some of the terms you'll find in this book

Sets and reps

Each time you perform an exercise – for example, when you lower and raise a barbell during a biceps curl – you have done one repetition, or 'rep'. A set is a series of reps performed back-to-back.

The plans in this book tell you how many sets and reps to perform of each exercise. So if the plan says '3 sets, 10-12 reps, 60 secs rest', then you'll do the exercise 10-12 times, rest for 60 seconds and then repeat two more times.

Failure

This is a technical term meaning the point at which you can no longer perform an exercise without breaking good form. For most exercises you should aim to reach failure at or near the stated rep range. So if you are required to do 10-12 reps of an exercise, choose a weight that allows you to complete all your reps, but no more.

Core

Your core muscles are those around your midriff, including your abs and lower back. They protect your spine and form the connection between your upper and lower body. Keeping your core engaged during heavy lifts will protect you from injury and help you lift more efficiently. To do this, imagine someone is about to punch you in the stomach and you are bracing for the impact. Maintain that contraction for the duration of your lift.

Concentric/eccentric

The lowering and lifting parts of an exercise are known as concentric and eccentric portions. Concentric is when the muscle shortens under tension, such as when you raise the barbell during a biceps curl. The eccentric portion is when the muscle lengthens under tension, such as the lowering part of a biceps curl.

Tempo

This is the speed at which you should perform your exercises, and is denoted in the workout guides by three numbers. The first number is for the eccentric (lowering) portion of the lift, which tends to be done quite slowly; the second number is the time you should take to pause before lifting; and the third number is the time you take to perform the concentric (lifting) portion of the exercise. For example, a tempo of '311' means you lower the weight over three seconds, pause for a second, then take one second to lift the weight again.

When you see the letter 'X', this means that the lift should be performed explosively, as fast as you can.

Intervals

This is a training method where you mix short bursts of intense activity with periods of recovery. For example, when running you might go as fast as possible for 30 seconds, then run slowly for two minutes before repeating the pattern several times. It's an intensive, but highly effective, way of increasing fitness and burning fat.

RPE

This stands for 'rating of perceived exertion' and it's used as a way of indicating the amount of effort you should use during the cardio training sessions: The higher the RPE, the harder you need to run, cycle, swim etc. For every cardio workout the RPE level is indicated as a number from 1-10 as follows:

1-3   Easy, up to a gentle pace
4-5   Faster, but still able to
      hold a conversation
6-7   Getting out of breath
8-9   Can't talk, uncomfortable
10   Flat-out sprint

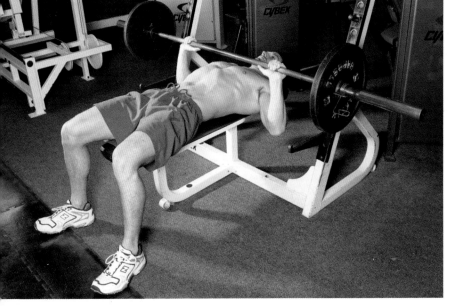

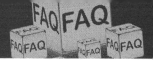

KNOW YOUR MUSCLES

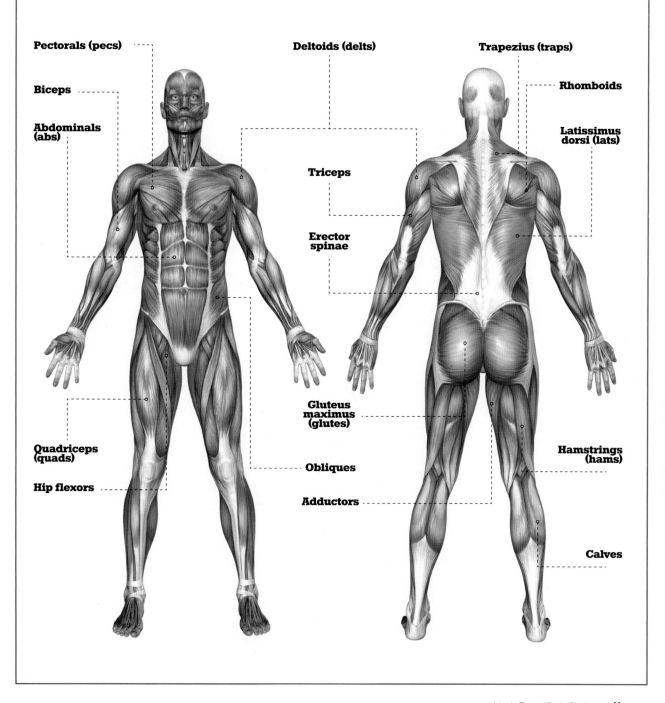

Pectorals (pecs)

Biceps

Abdominals
(abs)

Deltoids (delts)

Triceps

Erector
spinae

Trapezius (traps)

Rhomboids

Latissimus
dorsi (lats)

Gluteus
maximus
(glutes)

Obliques

Adductors

Quadriceps
(quads)

Hip flexors

Hamstrings
(hams)

Calves

Pre-workout stretches

Do this routine before every workout to prepare your body and prevent injury

Pre-workout warm-up

A proper warm-up is vital before doing any weight training. If time is short, don't be tempted to skip the warm-up and go straight to your workout, because cold muscles can get easily damaged. A few minutes saved on a warm-up can mean days lost while recovering from injury.

Your warm-up should start with some light cardiovascular exercise, such as running, rowing or cycling. This will make your heart beat faster, pumping oxygen and nutrients to your muscles, and elevating your body's core temperature. Warm muscles are more elastic than cold ones, which allows you to work them through a greater range of motion with less injury.

After the cardio you then need to target your muscles directly with dynamic stretches. These differ from static stretches in that you are moving as you stretch out the muscle (see examples opposite). The trick is to start very gently and then slowly increase the range of motion you use with each repetition. This prepares your muscles and joints for the work to come.

Finally, before you begin any lifting exercise, perform the movements with minimal weight to teach your muscles how to respond when you do the exercise with full weights.

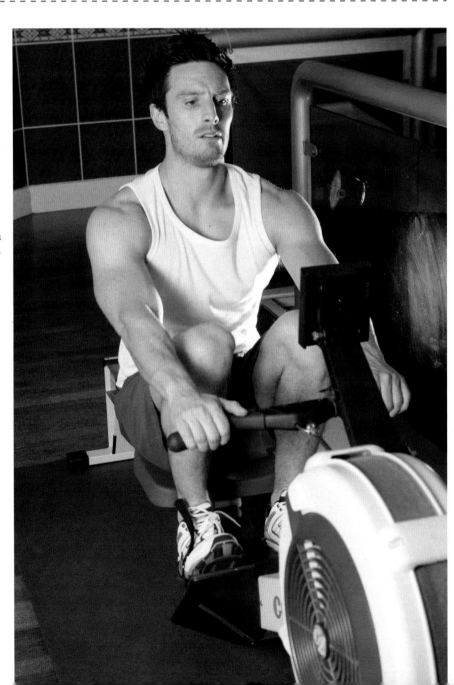

Cardio: 10 minutes

Whatever method of cardio warm-up you choose, keep the pace gentle and constant. By the end of ten minutes you should be sweating and puffing a bit, but not out of breath.

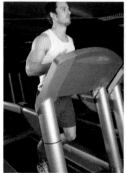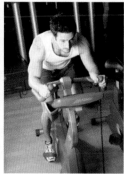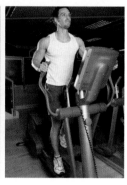

Dynamic stretches: 10 reps of each

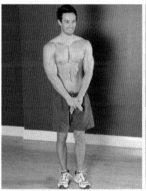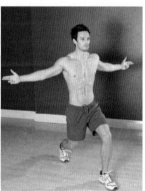

❶ Lunge with reverse flye

- Step forward while stretching your arms to the sides.
- Keep your body upright.
- Lunge lower with each rep.

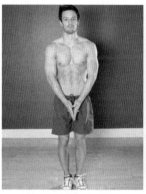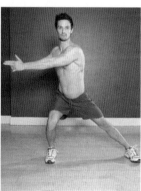

❷ Lateral lunge with twist

- Step to the side with both feet pointing forward.
- Twist your torso in the direction of your leading foot.
- Bend your knee a bit further with each rep.

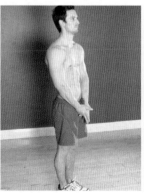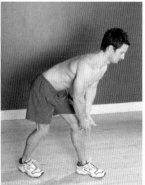

❸ Alternating split deadlift

- Step forward with one foot and lean forwards at the hips.
- Keep your back straight.
- Lower hands down a shin, a bit further each time, before pushing back to start.

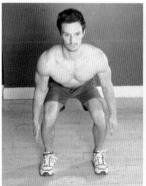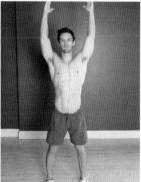

❹ Squat to overhead reach

- Feet shoulder width apart and back straight.
- Squat down and then reach overhead as you stand up.
- Squat a bit lower with each rep.

Post-workout stretches
Ease your tired muscles after every workout

Static stretches are where you hold a muscle under tension while relaxing it in order to lengthen the muscle after it has contracted as a result of weight training. Performing static stretches after a workout provides several benefits. First, it will help with flexibility, so you'll be able to work your muscles across a greater range of motion, leading to better muscle gains. Stretching also helps reduce injuries because your muscles and tendons are less likely to tear when they are relaxed.

Stretching improves blood flow to your muscles, helping to flush out toxins, meaning you'll be ready for your next workout earlier. And stretching can also aid posture, because tense muscles can pull your spine, shoulders and hips out of alignment, leading to a stooped look and lower-back pain.

Your muscles need to be fully warmed up before performing static stretches, so never do them at the beginning of a workout. Also, to avoid injury, don't pull too hard when you stretch, and don't 'bounce' the muscle under tension.

Static stretches: hold each for 20-30 seconds

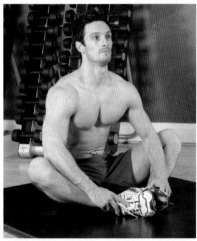

Adductors
● Press your knees apart gently with your elbows.

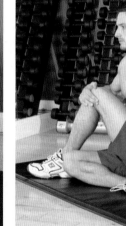

Glutes
● Gently pull on your knee.

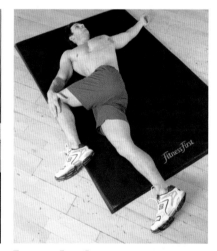

Lower back
● Keep your shoulders flat on the floor.

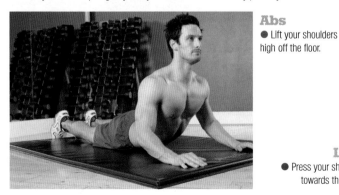

Abs
● Lift your shoulders high off the floor.

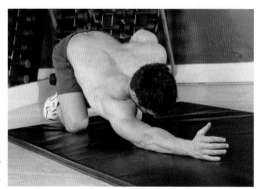

Lats
● Press your shoulder towards the floor.

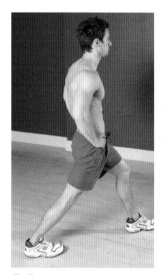

Calves
● Push down on your rear heel until you feel the pull in your calf muscle.

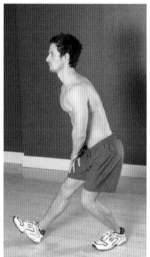

Hamstrings
● Lean forward at the hips with a straight back.

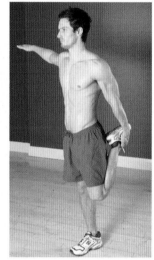

Quads
● Pull on your ankle and push your hips forward.

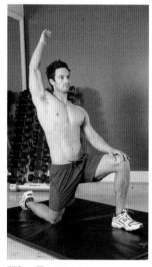

Hip flexors
● Keep your body upright and push your hips forward.

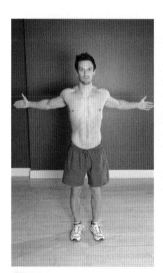

Chest
● Press your hands backwards with straight arms.

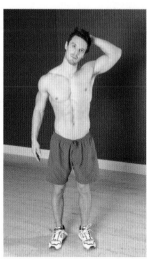

Traps
● Pull gently on your head until you feel the pull in your shoulder muscle.

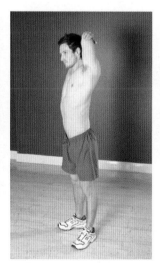

Triceps
● Point your fingers down your back and pull gently on your elbow.

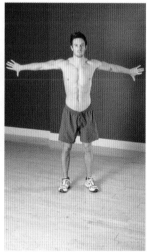

Biceps
● Press arms back and twist hands so your thumbs point behind you.

Make every rep count
Follow these tips to get the most from your workouts

Stay positive

Getting into the right frame of mind can make a massive difference to the effectiveness of your workouts. On your way to the gym, remind yourself of all the reasons why you started the plan, and think about how good you'll feel when you reach your goals. You'll be far more likely to work harder if you're not simply going through the motions.

If you're having an off day, and don't feel like training, go anyway, get changed and do a light warm-up. The surge of feel-good hormones may make you change your mind about skipping a session. And if you do miss a session, don't get discouraged. Simply pick up where you left off at the next workout.

Keep your core tight

Before any heavy lift, tighten your core muscles – those around your midriff – to protect your lower back from injury. Don't be tempted to compensate for weak abs by using a weight-lifter's belt. It's better to pick a lighter weight and build up slowly as your core strength increases.

Pick the right weight

The right weight is one you can control properly, and that allows you to complete all your reps – but no more – with perfect form. Too many men pick a weight that they struggle to handle, risking injury. However, if you choose a weight that you can manage too easily, your muscles won't get enough stimulation to grow.

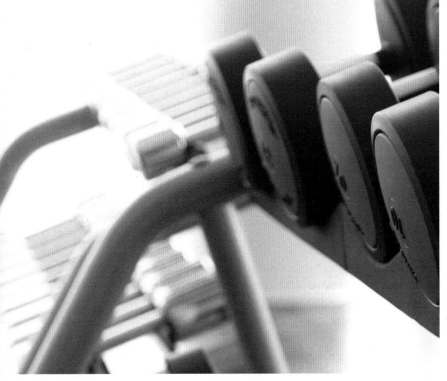

Don't forget to breathe

Never hold your breath during a heavy lift. Instead the general rule is to breathe in as you lower the weight, and breathe out through pursed lips as you lift the weight.

If it hurts – stop!

Pain is your body's way of telling you something is wrong. If you feel pain at any time, stop immediately and don't resume training until you are fully recovered. Seek medical help if you are unsure whether you should train or not.

Time your sets

Each set should take you around 40-45 seconds to complete. Any faster and you're not putting your muscles under tension long enough to get good results. Therefore, each rep should take three or four seconds. Make the lowering (eccentric) portion of the lift slow and controlled, and then move powerfully through the exertion (concentric) part of the lift.

Get some balance

To ensure that your muscle growth is even across your body, aim to make your workouts as balanced as possible. This means that you should do as many lower-body moves as upper-body; for every pushing motion you should do a pulling one; and you give the same amount of attention to opposing muscle groups, such as biceps and triceps. Following this plan will give you the right balance but, if you have one side of your body stronger than the other, work your weaker side harder to help it catch up.

Be progressive

Aim to increase the resistance you use for an exercise by around 10 per cent every three to four weeks. This will ensure that your muscles get the stimulation they need to grow. If the weights don't get bigger neither will your muscles.

Mind your manners

There are a few unwritten rules of gym etiquette that you should follow if you don't want to be ostracised by your fellow gym members. Never hog a machine or a piece of equipment. Wipe your sweat off any equipment after you've used it. Replace dumbbells and weight plates on their racks after you've used them. Don't trail water from the showers into the changing rooms. And don't ogle the girlfriend of the guy who's bench pressing 200kg.

Stay hydrated

Most gyms provide water, but take a bottle with you so you can sip from it every few minutes to keep your water levels topped up. If you wait until you're thirsty before drinking, you'll probably already be dehydrated and your performance will suffer as a result.

Try something new

Many men stick to the same workout week-in and week-out. If you always do the same workout your body will adapt to it and stop growing new muscle. Keep altering your workout every few weeks, even if that simply means using different items of equipment, or changing the angle on your bench, or altering the order you perform the exercises in. Change is good for your muscles.

Get your rest

Your muscles don't grow in the gym. They grow while they are recovering afterwards. That's why you shouldn't train the same muscle groups two days in a row, because they won't have had time to repair themselves from the first workout by the time you hit them again. If you want more muscle, always take rest days and make sure you get enough sleep.

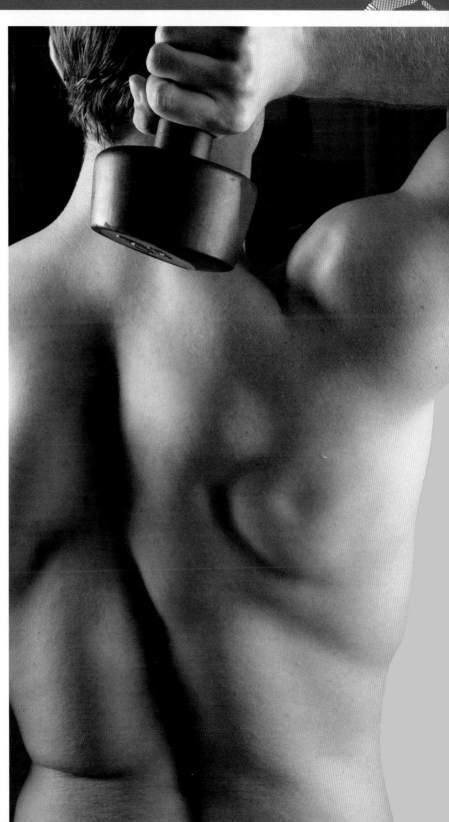

Eat for a better body

Good nutrition is half the battle, so follow these basic rules and start seeing a real change to your body

1 Watch your calories

Put simply, if you eat fewer calories each day than you burn off through activity you will lose weight. If you eat more, you'll gain weight. Of course, whether you gain that weight as fat or muscle will depend on the kind of foods you eat and the training you do.

For the *Body Challenge* programme you'll eat between 2,500 and 3,000 calories a day. The average man needs around 2,500 calories a day just to sustain himself, so the extra will go towards fuelling your workouts and building new muscle.

2 Get the balance right

Nearly all your calories come from a combination of carbohydrates, protein and fats. Carbohydrates provide the muscle glycogen that fuels your workouts and should make up about 50-60 per cent of your total calorie intake.

Protein is required to grow new tissue in your body and is therefore of particular interest to anyone building muscle. The optimum intake of protein for muscle-gainers is between 1.5g and 2g of protein per kilo of bodyweight, but it doesn't hurt to take in a bit more to ensure that you are hitting your daily protein targets.

Fat is a nutrient that many people try to avoid altogether, but it will help you absorb vitamins, improve athletic performance and protect joints and tendons against injury. However fat is a very energy-dense nutrient, containing nine calories per gram compared to four calories for carbs and protein, so you only need about 50-60g of fat a day.

3 Eat the right stuff

The simplest rule when deciding what to eat is: keep it natural. Processed foods – biscuits, cakes, ready meals, fizzy drinks, crisps – tend to be high in calories but low on essential nutrients, so they are poor at fuelling workouts and rebuilding muscle but good at making you fat and sapping your energy.

Carbohydrates provide the energy you need to train hard, but they can also be responsible for altering your blood sugar levels and making you store fat, so the simplest rule to follow is to make the majority of your carbs unrefined, unprocessed, low on the glycaemic index and high in fibre. This includes wholewheat bread and pasta, oats, beans, fruit and vegetables. These will release energy slowly, ensuring you always have enough stored glycogen in your muscles for a workout.

Protein-rich foods include lean meat, fish, eggs, dairy produce and soya. Lower-quality protein can also be found in nuts, seeds and beans. Aim to eat a wide variety of protein foods to get the full range of muscle-building amino acids, but be wary of taking in too much saturated fat, such as can be found in poor cuts of red meat and dairy items.

Fats are not all bad. The ones to avoid are saturates and trans fats, which means skipping cakes, biscuits and margarine and cutting back on red meats and cheese. The fats you need are monounsaturates and polyunsaturates, found in olive oil, nuts, seeds and oily fish. These include omega 3 and omega 6 fatty acids, which have been proven to aid strength and aerobic training and protect the body from injuries.

4 Eat at the right times

When you're training hard you want to eat about an hour or two before your workouts, and again immediately afterwards. Your snacks should include both carbs and protein to help restore glycogen levels in your muscles and repair muscle tissue. A perfect post-workout snack might be a bagel with cream cheese, or a tuna and pasta salad.

For the rest of the day, eat small meals at regular intervals of two or three hours, with the aim of having some protein with every meal. This way you keep your glycogen levels topped up and prevent your body from breaking down the proteins that you need for muscle rebuilding.

5 Take on fluids – but not booze

When you work out you sweat a lot, and you need to replace that fluid with water. The trick is to ensure that you hydrate yourself before you get thirsty, not afterwards. Dehydration will impact on your performance in the gym and can affect the way your body stores fat and repairs muscle owing to poor organ function. Take a water bottle with you to the gym and sip from it every few minutes. Over the course of a day you should aim to take in about three litres of water in total.

Alcohol, on the other hand, you can do without. It can have a catabolic effect on your muscles, meaning it prevents them from developing properly.

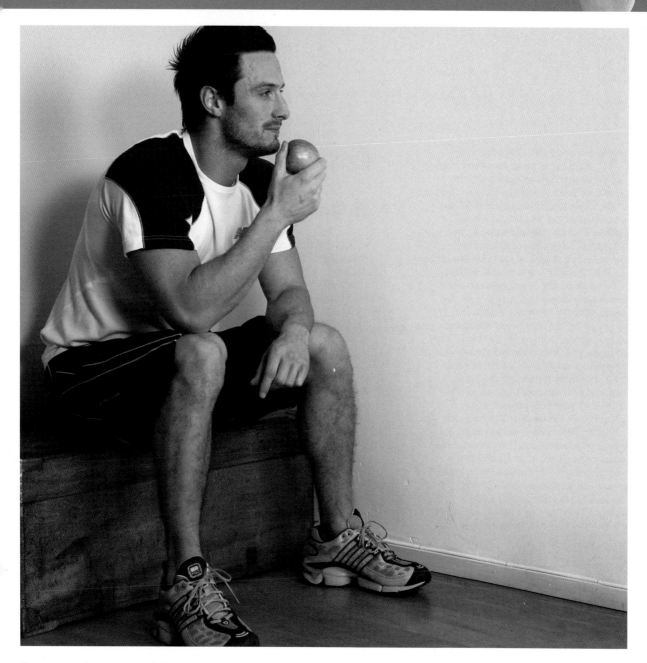

If you are serious about gaining muscle mass, keep your sessions in the pub to a minimum.

6 Should you take supplements?

Sports supplements, such as protein powders and energy drinks, shouldn't be seen as an alternative to a good diet. Eating healthily is more important than glugging down shakes, but they do have one advantage: convenience. It can be tough to consume all the calories you need every day through food alone, and it's much easier to take a protein shake to the gym that to whip up a chicken salad, so supplements can be useful. Also, people who do a lot of exercise can need extra vitamins C and E, so a supplement of these can be handy if you struggle to get enough in your diet.

If you do use supplements, be sure to pick a reputable brand and follow the guidelines on the packaging.

On your plate

Great meals to feed your muscles and torch your fat

The *Body Challenge* comes with meal plans for every day of the 12-week programme. However, it's not always easy to stick to these plans, especially if you have a busy lifestyle. You might not be able to find all the ingredients; you might not have time to prepare all the meals; it might be that you simply don't like some of the foods on offer.

Not a problem. If you can't stick to the meal plans exactly, then you can adapt them to suit your needs. Just try to eat a similar number of calories each day, and aim to eat the same kind of foods you see on the meal plan (no swapping a salad for a burger and fries, now). By following the basic rules of nutrition, as laid out on p18-19, you should still be able to see great results at the end of 12 weeks.

To help you along, we've created a range of healthy and tasty breakfasts, lunches, dinners and snacks that you can use to create your own meal plans. Each of them will provide the nutrients and vitamins you need to burn fat and build muscle during the 12-week programme.

Breakfast

① Strawberry smoothie

WHAT YOU'LL NEED

20 strawberries
50g oats
350ml milk
1tbsp flaxseed oil

TO MAKE

● Mix all the ingredients together. Blend and serve chilled.

WHY YOU SHOULD HAVE IT

● Flaxseed oil has a large amount of healthy fat, which reduces inflammation and builds bone mass
● Oats contain fibre and slow-release carbs that'll give you long-lasting energy.

● Milk supplies B vitamins, which helps turn food into energy and protein for building and maintaining muscle.
● The vitamin C and flavonoids from the strawberries will protect cells and tissue from free radicals.

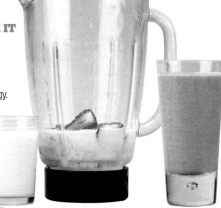

Snacks

HANDFUL OF PECAN NUTS

● As well as being particularly tasty, pecans are high in protein and antioxidants and are loaded with oleic acid, a type of good fat that supports the muscle-building hormone testosterone.

PEANUT BUTTER ON OATCAKES

● The oakcakes' roughage will fill you up, while peanut butter contains protein, iron and magnesium, which are all needed to build muscle.

LOW-FAT YOGHURT TOPPED WITH OATS AND BLUEBERRIES

● Yoghurt and oats are a good source of protein and calcium both of which are needed for fuelling muscles, while the blueberries are packed with antioxidants, which will help you fight off the damaging free radicals that are produced during exercise.

FRESH BERRIES

● Loaded with antioxidants, berries will keep your immune system strong. They are also packed with vitamin C, which helps our body to absorb iron from plant foods.

EDAMAME BEANS

● Also known as soyabeans, they are one of the few vegetable sources of all eight essential amino acids (the protein

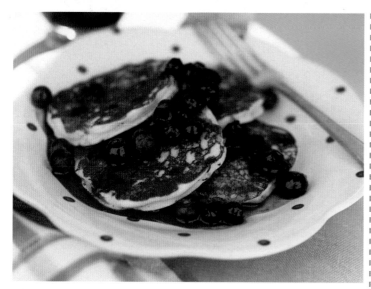

② Protein pancakes

WHAT YOU'LL NEED
150g pancake mix
Water (see pancake mix packet for amount)
50g whey protein
100g cottage cheese
3 eggs (1 whole, 2 whites)
Handful of blueberries

TO MAKE
● Blend the egg, cottage cheese and water in a blender until smooth. Pour the ingredients into a bowl, mix with the pancake mix and protein powder and then add the blueberries. Heat a frying pan coated with olive oil and pour in the pancake mix to the thickness of 3mm. Once the pancakes start to solidify and brown on the underside, flip the pancakes to lightly brown them.

WHY YOU SHOULD HAVE THEM
● As well as being low in fat, eggs are packed with protein and will stock your body with a good balance of the amino acids needed for muscle growth.
● Cottage cheese is a low-fat source of protein that fuels muscles. It is also packed with calcium, which initiates muscle growth and transmits nerve signals in the muscles.
● Blueberries are extremely rich in disease-fighting antioxidants.
● Whey protein will help your muscles repair and grow, as well as aid satiety.

③ Power porridge

WHAT YOU'LL NEED
45g oats
1 chopped banana
Handful of muesli
Glass of semi skimmed milk
Sprinkle of cinnamon

TO MAKE
● Mix the oats with the milk and heat in a saucepan until hot. Chop up the banana and stir into the bowl along with a handful of muesli and a sprinkle of cinnamon to taste.

WHY YOU SHOULD HAVE IT
● Oats have a low glycaemic index (GI), which will give you a steady flow of energy throughout the morning.
● Bananas are stuffed with fibre to keep you feeling full. Their natural sugar content will also curb any sweet cravings and supply a natural, sustained release of energy all day long.
● Milk is full of calcium, which helps support bone health and protein, which helps build and repair muscles.
● The seeds in the muesli will help improve blood flow to your muscles during exercise and transport fat to where it can be used as energy.
● Cinnamon helps the cells absorb glucose more efficiently, making energy levels consistent, and can also lower cholesterol.

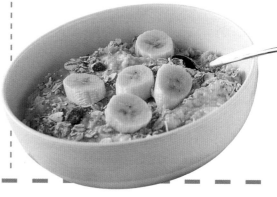

molecules that the body can't make itself) and are a near complete protein. They are also rich in iron, which is essential for transporting oxygen to muscles.

BANANAS
● Bananas are an ideal post-exercise snack. They contain natural sugars for sustained energy and plenty of fibre. They're also rich in vitamin B6, which regulates blood sugar levels, and are a good source of potassium, which helps prevent muscle fatigue.

SUNFLOWER SEEDS
● Seeds contain vitamin E and zinc, which can have a positive effect on your testosterone levels. They also provide a generous helping of muscle-building protein and selenium, a powerful antioxidant that will help fight off free-radical damage and aid recovery.

DRIED APRICOTS
● They contain immunity-boosting betacarotene, calcium for proper nerve and muscle function, and potassium, which supports muscle contraction and glycogen storage.

CHOCOLATE MILK
● According to researchers at Indiana University, drinking chocolate milk after a workout will boost muscle growth and speed recovery. This is down to its high quality combination of protein and carbs.

HUMMUS AND CARROTS
● Hummus contains iron to keep energy levels up and vitamin E needed for muscle stamina. Combine with raw carrots, which provide a handy dose of potassium to regulate the body's fluid levels.

Lunches

1 Egg and tomato bagel

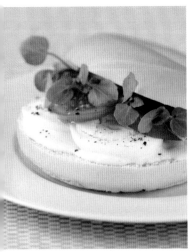

WHAT YOU'LL NEED
1 white bagel, halved
3tbsp low-fat mayonnaise
mixed with 1tbsp Dijon mustard
1 hard-boiled egg, sliced
1 tomato, chopped
1tbsp watercress
Black pepper

TO MAKE
● Spread the mustard mayonnaise on each side of the bagel. Layer the rest of the ingredients and finish with a seasoning of black pepper.

WHY YOU SHOULD HAVE IT
● Eggs contain all eight of the essential amino acids that your hard-working muscles need to build and repair themselves.
● Weight for weight, watercress has more energy-promoting iron than spinach and more bone-building calcium than milk.
● The vitamin C in tomatoes makes a hefty contribution to your amino acid metabolism, which helps the body form new muscle.
● Mustard ups blood flow to muscles, while mayonnaise contains vitamin E, a powerful antioxidant that neutralises cancer-causing free radicals.
● Bagels are a high-GI carbohydrate, meaning its glucose enters your bloodstream fast and drives the protein from the egg into your muscles.

2 Bean salad

WHAT YOU'LL NEED
1 small onion, chopped
1 red pepper, chopped
1tbsp olive oil
200g can of mixed beans
½ lemon
1tsp chopped parsley
Handful of watercress
Handful of iceberg lettuce
1tbsp grated cheese
Black pepper

TO MAKE
● Heat the olive oil in a small pan and fry the onion and pepper on a medium heat for three minutes. Drain and rinse the mixed beans, add to the pan and cook for another minute, stirring. Remove the pan from the heat and add the juice of half a lemon and parsley. Stir and leave to cool.
● Place the watercress and iceberg lettuce in a separate container and toss together. Place the bean mixture on top of this and finish off with a pinch of black pepper and grated cheese.

WHY YOU SHOULD HAVE IT
● Watercress is full of calcium and magnesium. It's also virtually calorie-free so you can eat plenty without needing to loosen your belt.
● The folate in the onions works with the vitamin C from the peppers, helping you digest and use the protein from the beans and cheese.
● Beans are bursting with protein and fall low on the GI index, which means their carbohydrates are broken down to glucose and absorbed more slowly. This makes them a slow-release, long-lasting energy supply.
● Parsley is full of fatigue-fighting iron – needed for the production of haemoglobin, which carries oxygen from the lungs to the muscles.

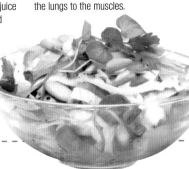

3 Honey and ham baguette

WHAT YOU'LL NEED
1 wholemeal baguette
1tbsp honey
½ green apple
2 slices cooked ham
Grated low-fat cheddar

TO MAKE
● Cut a wholemeal baguette in half and spread evenly with honey. Cut half a green apple into thin slices. Layer the cooked ham in the baguette with the green apple strips and top with a layer of grated low-fat cheddar.

WHY YOU SHOULD HAVE IT
● Ham is a good source of slow-absorbing protein, which helps build and repair muscle.

● The baguette will provide you with a good source of fibre and slow-release carbs, keeping your gut healthy and satisfied.
● Honey is a natural energy food that boosts your immune system.
● The water from the apple will help to rehydrate your body. The mineral boron, which is also found in the fruit, will build strong bones.
● Cheese works with the carbs from the bread to speed up glycogen replenishment, as well as supplying protein to promote muscle growth and restoration.

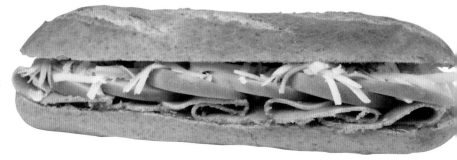

Dinners

① The muscle pot

WHAT YOU'LL NEED
225g lean shoulder of pork, diced
2tbsp light soy sauce
Sprinkle of sugar
½ clove garlic, chopped
½ chilli, chopped
30ml sherry
300ml stock
4 salad potatoes
1 spring onion, chopped
100g spinach leaves
Salt and freshly ground pepper to taste

TO MAKE
● Arrange the pork in the base of a lidded casserole dish. Mix the sugar, soy sauce, garlic and chillies with the sherry and stock, stir well and pour over the pork. Add the veg, then place the casserole on the hob and bring it to a gentle simmer. Put the lid on and simmer over a gentle heat for 90 minutes, stirring occasionally.

WHY YOU SHOULD HAVE IT
● Potatoes will keep your glycogen levels topped up, so your body doesn't use your protein stores for fuel.
● Pork provides plenty of muscle-building protein and is brimming with magnesium, which helps keep muscles strong.
● Spinach is rich in vitamin C, folate and betacarotene – all needed for a healthy immune system – as well as supplying iron and calcium.
● Black pepper helps the stomach produce hydrochloric acid, making it easier to digest your food.

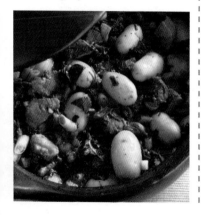

② Chicken and mushroom pasta

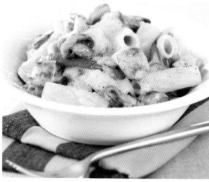

TO MAKE
● Heat oil in a pan and cook the onion and pepper for five minutes. Add the chicken and brown, then add the mushrooms and continue cooking for five minutes. Remove from heat and stir in the fromage frais. Meanwhile, cook the pasta according to packet instructions. Drain and combine with the chicken and mushroom mix. Top with cheddar and place under the grill until the cheese is golden brown and crispy.

WHY YOU SHOULD HAVE IT
● Onions are rich in chromium, which helps fight fat by regulating blood sugar levels.
● The carbs in pasta will help your muscles recover and top up your glycogen stores.
● Fromage frais contains muscle-friendly protein and calcium, which helps prevent fat storage.
● Chicken is bursting with protein and zinc, two key nutrients needed to boost testosterone and muscle growth.
● Mushrooms are rich in riboflavin, which is essential for the release of energy from carbohydrate.

WHAT YOU'LL NEED
1tsp olive oil
½ onion, sliced
½ green pepper, sliced
1 chicken breast, chopped
50g mushrooms, sliced
1tbsp fromage frais
60g pasta
1tsp cheddar

③ Muscle burritos

WHAT YOU'LL NEED
3 egg whites
¼ tsp black pepper
28g low-fat cottage cheese
2 wholemeal tortillas
15g mushrooms, sliced
¼ onion chopped
1 red pepper, diced
Grated low-fat cheese
Salsa

TO MAKE
● Whisk together the egg white, pepper, and cottage cheese. Place the tortillas in a low oven to warm through. Lightly coat a medium saucepan with low-fat cooking spray and place over medium high heat. Sauté the mushrooms, onion and red pepper until soft. Pour the egg mixture over the vegetables and cook until it is firm. Place a small amount of the egg and vegetable mixture down the centre of each warm tortilla. Roll each up and then top with some grated low-fat cheese and salsa.

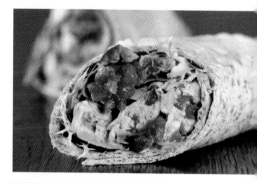

WHY YOU SHOULD HAVE IT
● Cottage cheese is a low-calorie source of riboflavin, a micronutrient vital for muscle growth and blood cell production, and high-quality protein.
● Mushrooms are high in the hydrating mineral potassium, which also helps convert sugar into energy-providing glycogen.
● Wholemeal tortillas have a medium GI, which combined with the protein in the meal helps slow down carbohydrate absorption even more.
● Peppers will provide you with a good dose of vitamin C to help boost your immune system.

WEEK 1
GETTING STABILISED

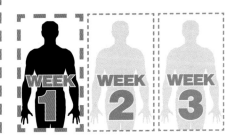

WEEK 1 WEEK 2 WEEK 3

The first week is all about getting your muscles used to training. Before you can start lifting heavy weights you need to teach your body how to stabilise itself, which means doing exercises that strengthen your joints and core muscles – the ones around your midriff that protect your spine.

For beginners, this provides a gentle introduction to training, but even if you are experienced at weight training, don't skip this stage in the 12-week plan because it forms the foundation upon which you'll build later on.

The most important thing to concentrate on this week is getting the form correct for each exercise. Pick a light weight, take everything slow and make all your movements controlled. If you feel pain at any time, stop immediately and rest.

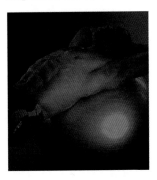

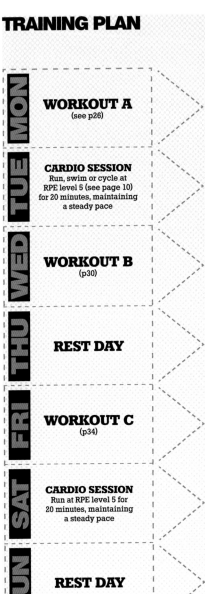

TRAINING PLAN

MON
WORKOUT A
(see p26)

TUE
CARDIO SESSION
Run, swim or cycle at RPE level 5 (see page 10) for 20 minutes, maintaining a steady pace

WED
WORKOUT B
(p30)

THU
REST DAY

FRI
WORKOUT C
(p34)

SAT
CARDIO SESSION
Run at RPE level 5 for 20 minutes, maintaining a steady pace

SUN
REST DAY

MEAL PLAN

Breakfast	Snack
Scramble 2 egg yolks and 5 whites. Serve on 4 slices wholemeal toast with tomato ketchup.	1 bowl of granola with 110g blueberries, 225g low-fat natural yoghurt and 1 apple. Glass of semi-skimmed milk.
100g muesli with 250g natural yoghurt. 1 pomegranate.	30g walnuts. 1 apple.
2 slices of rye bread with 1 sliced avocado. 100g muesli with 150ml whole milk. 250ml cranberry juice.	250g flapjack
Porridge made with 100g oats, 500ml skimmed milk and 40g mixed nuts. 250ml pressed apple juice.	Protein shake made with 500ml semi-skimmed milk.
2 slices of rye bread with 1 sliced avocado and 1 sliced tomato. 250ml fresh orange juice.	Smoothie: blend 1 banana, 125g strawberries, 1tbsp honey and 425ml whole milk.
1 plain bagel with 5 scrambled egg whites and 50g smoked salmon.	1 apple. 33g cereal bar.
2 poached eggs, small tin of baked beans, 2 grilled tomatoes, 4 rashers lean bacon and 2 slices wholemeal toast.	Blend 1½ bananas and 1 scoop of whey protein powder with 500ml water.

WEEK 4 **WEEK 5** **WEEK 6** **WEEK 7** **WEEK 8** **WEEK 9** **WEEK 10** **WEEK 11** **WEEK 12**

Lunch	Snack	Dinner	Snack	Total
1 wholemeal bagel with 1tbsp peanut butter and 225g cottage cheese.	Raisin, cranberry and almond snack bar.	Sprinkle a dash of pepper, a squeeze of lemon and 1tbsp grated Parmesan over 115g rainbow trout. Place in tinfoil with a chopped onion and bake at 180°C/Gas Mark 4 for 20-30 minutes. Stir-fry 200g broccoli florets with a clove of crushed garlic. Serve with 50g brown rice.	150g strawberries.	**2,848 calories** 163g protein 401g carbs 77g fat
200g roast lamb, 100g steamed broccoli, 75g steamed green beans and 75g parsnips roasted in 2tbsp avocado oil.	4 wholemeal oat crackers with pâté. 1 peach.	Grill 115g salmon with 15g butter and a slice of lemon on top. Serve with 1 mashed sweet potato and salad (100g lettuce, 1 sliced radish and a handful of water cress drizzled with balsamic vinegar).	1 slice of wholemeal toast spread with peanut butter.	**2,995 calories** 226g protein 390g carbs 59g fat
150g chicken with 100g mixed salad leaves and 25g cubed feta cheese. Sprinkle with a handful of mixed seeds and drizzle with olive oil.	Smoothie: blend 1 mango, 1 passion fruit, 300ml whole milk and 30g oats.	200g grilled steak served with 150g steamed broccoli and 150g steamed cauliflower. Sprinkle vegetables with 20g grated cheese and a few sesame seeds.	30g almonds.	**2,957 calories** 227g protein 402g carbs 49g fat
6 fish fingers served on wholemeal pitta bread.	1 orange. 2 bananas.	Place a 250g mackerel fillet in a foil parcel. Cover in garlic cloves, the juice of 1 lemon and a little basil. Cook at 200°C/Gas Mark 6 for 20 minutes. Serve with a medium jacket potato and 30g of low-fat coleslaw.	125g low-fat yoghurt.	**2,520 calories** 169g protein 390g carbs 57g fat
Dice and grill 1 carrot, 1 red pepper and 1 red onion. Mix with 75g couscous, 1tbsp coconut oil and 30g cashew nuts.	4 wholemeal oat crackers with 100g thin smoked salmon and 25g grated cheese.	115g grilled mackerel placed on 75g brown rice. Pour over a sauce made with tinned tomatoes and 1 chopped leek.	30g walnuts.	**2,965 calories** 210g protein 412g carbs 53g fat
1 medium baked potato with 100g tuna in brine and a handful of mixed salad leaves.	Protein shake made with 500ml semi-skimmed milk.	Home-made pizza: top an 8in pizza base with 200g passata and ½tsp dried oregano, 65g low-fat cheddar cheese, 100g turkey, cooked, 25g salami 30g chillies, and a splash of Tabasco sauce.	1 apple and 25g almonds.	**2,505 calories** 156g protein 375g carbs 53g fat
Tuna salad sandwich: ½ tin tuna, 110g diced celery, 2tbsp mayonnaise, 1tbsp lemon juice, 2 leaves iceberg lettuce and a few slices cucumber on 2 slices wholemeal bread.	220g low-fat cottage cheese and 1tbsp peanut butter on an English muffin. 250ml orange juice.	Glazed pork chop: cook a 115g lean centre-cut pork chop until meat is white. Mix 1tsp of mustard, 2tbsp sugar, ½tsp of cinnamon and ½tsp of basil and place on the chop. Return the chop to the oven until top is brown. Serve with 50g rice and 4 steamed baby carrots.	½ tin sliced peaches.	**2,057 calories** 202g protein 345g carbs 74g fat

WORKOUT A

For your first workout, remember to keep the weights light and your movements slow and controlled.

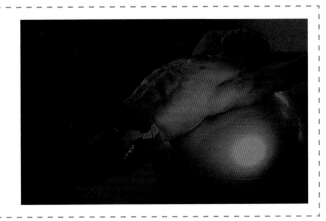

Warm-up Ten minutes of gentle cardio followed by dynamic stretches (see p13)

Exercise		Sets	Reps	Tempo	Rest	Weight
① Cuban press		2	12-15	313	30 secs	
② Dumb-bell squat		2	12-15	312	30 secs	
③ Two-point box		2	10 each side	121	30 secs	n/a
④ Gym ball static press-up		2	10-30 secs	n/a	30 secs	n/a
⑤ Standing cable Russian twist		2	12-15 each side	311	30 secs	
⑥ Side plank		1	20-30 secs each side	n/a	n/a	n/a

Warm down and stretch Ten minutes of gentle cardio plus static stretches (20 seconds each). Focus on quads, hams, lower back, upper back, chest, shoulders (see p14)

Notes

❶ Cuban press

Target: rotator cuff (internal shoulders), deltoids

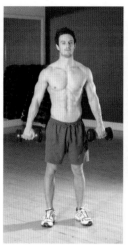 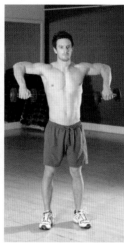 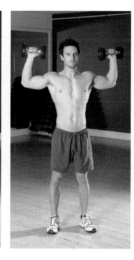 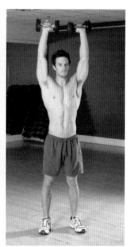

- With your core braced hold a pair of light dumb-bells by your sides, palms facing back.
- Lift your arms out to the sides until your elbows are at 90° and the weights hang straight down.

- Keeping your upper arms horizontal, rotate them until your hands point up.
- Press the weights directly overhead then reverse the movement back to the start.

❷ Dumb-bell squat

Target: quads, glutes, hamstrings

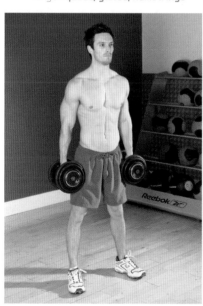 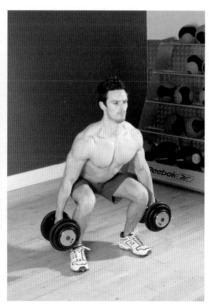

- Stand with your feet shoulder width apart, holding the dumb-bells by your sides.
- Brace your core and maintain a natural arch in your back throughout the movement.
- Keep your knees in line with your feet and lower until your thighs are parallel to the ground.
- Push back up through your heels.

③ Two-point box

Target: lower back

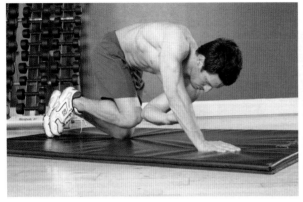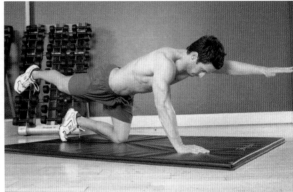

● Kneel on all fours and keep looking down throughout the movement.

● Bring one elbow to meet the opposite knee beneath your stomach before stretching out your arm and leg.

● Your body should form a straight line from foot to fingertip, don't let your hips rotate.

● Hold this position for a count of two, return to the start and repeat on the other side.

④ Gym ball static press-up

Target: pecs

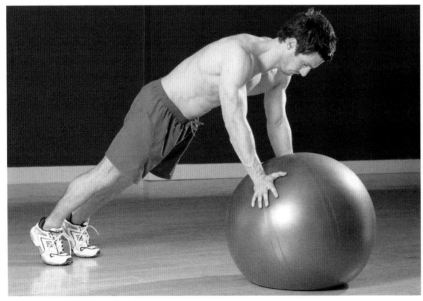

● Brace your core to keep your body in a straight line from head to heels.

● Grip the sides of the ball with your hands roughly in line with your shoulders.

● Hold this position for 10-30 seconds.

⑤ Standing cable Russian twist

Target: core, obliques

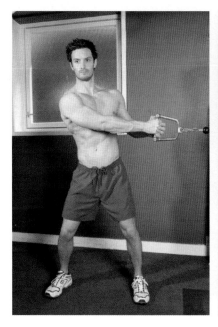
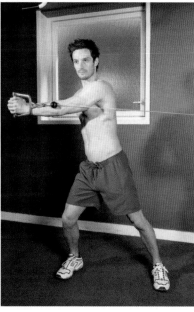

● Stand side-on to a cable machine set at chest height, core braced.

● With your arms straight and head facing forward, twist your torso away from the cable.

● Return to the start position with a slow and controlled motion.

⑥ Side plank

Target: core, obliques

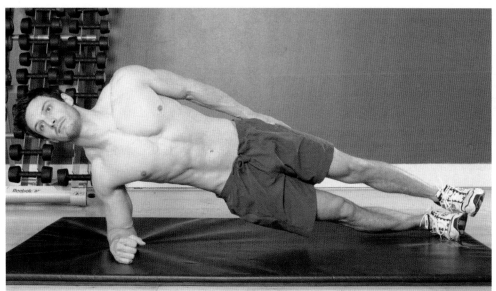

● With your elbow positioned directly below your shoulder, hold your body in a straight line from head to heels.

● Maintain this position for as long as you can without letting your hips drop, then repeat on the other side.

WORKOUT B

Focus on maintaining perfect form for all your movements. At this stage you are still teaching your body how to train, so don't over-stress it with heavy weights.

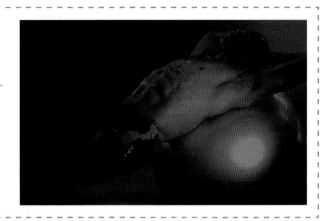

Warm-up Ten minutes of gentle cardio followed by dynamic stretches (see p13)

Exercise		Sets	Reps	Tempo	Rest	Weight
① Cable squat to overhead raise		2	12-15	312	30 secs	
② Close-grip pull down to triceps press down		2	12-15	312	30 secs	
③ Gym ball roll out		2	12-15	313	30 secs	n/a
④ Gym ball jackknife		2	10	212	30 secs	n/a
⑤ Gym ball hip raise and leg curl		2	10	313	30 secs	n/a
⑥ Plank		1	30-60 secs	n/a	n/a	n/a

Warm down and stretch Ten minutes of gentle cardio plus static stretches
(20 seconds each). Focus on quads, hams, glutes lower back, abs, lats, triceps, shoulders (see p14)

Notes

❶ Cable squat to overhead raise

Target: legs, shoulders, back, core

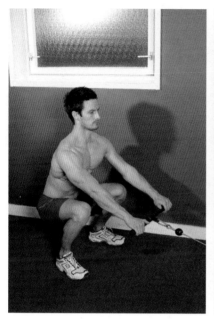 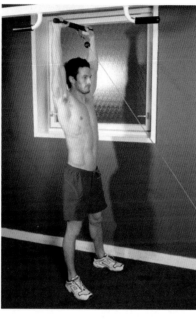

● Squat down facing a low cable, keep your back straight and your knees in line with your feet.

● Brace your core, drive up through your heels, lifting the handle overhead while keeping your arms straight.

● Reverse the movement in a controlled manner.

❷ Close-grip pull down to triceps press down

Target: lats, traps, rhomboids, triceps

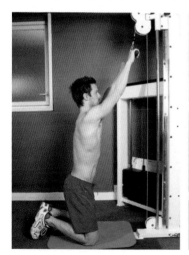 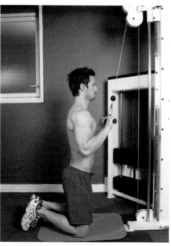 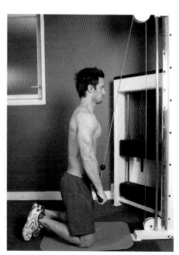

● Grip a short bar with your palms facing away from you.

● Keeping your body upright, retract your shoulder blades and pull your elbows into your sides.

● Press the bar down without moving your elbows or upper arms.

● Reverse the motion in a controlled manner.

③ Gym ball roll out

Target: core

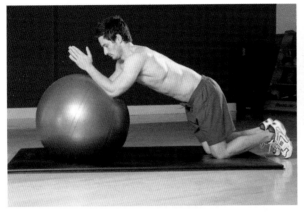 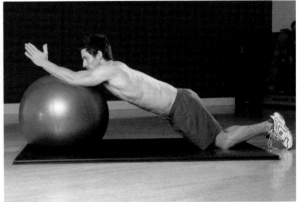

● Brace your core and rest your forearms on the ball just beneath your shoulders.

● Keep your back straight and use your abs to maintain a slow and steady pace, controlling any wobbling.

● Roll the ball out as far as you can without breaking form, then return.

④ Gym ball jackknife

Target: upper and lower abdominals

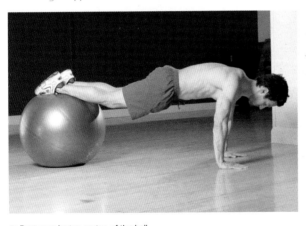 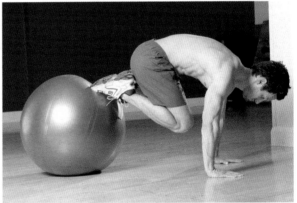

● Rest your instep on top of the ball with your body in a straight line and your hands directly beneath your shoulders.

● In a smooth controlled motion roll your feet over the ball to draw your knees into your chest while avoiding lifting your backside.

⑤ Gym ball hip raise and leg curl

Target: **hamstrings, hip flexors**

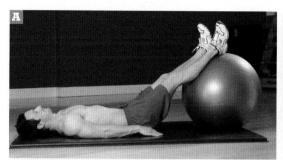

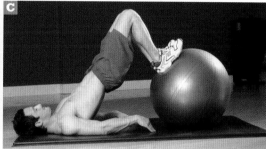

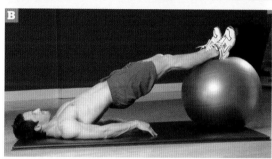

● Start with your body flat on the floor and your feet together, resting on top of the ball.

● Brace your core and raise your hips until your body forms a straight line from your shoulders to your heels.

● Roll the ball towards your backside with your heels, raising your hips to keep your body straight.

● Pause at the top of the movement and slowly return to the start.

⑥ Plank

Target: **core**

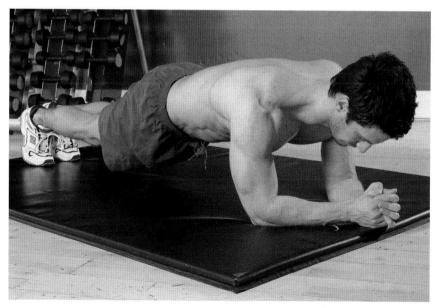

● Position yourself with your feet together and elbows directly beneath your shoulders so that your body is straight from head to heels.

● Keep your head looking down and hold that position for 30-60 seconds without letting your hips sag.

WORKOUT C

You may be feeling a bit stiff after the previous workouts, so start slowly and build up gently to ease your muscles back into action.

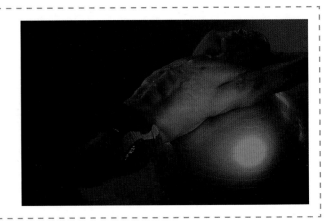

Warm-up Ten minutes of gentle cardio followed by dynamic stretches (see p13)

Exercise	Sets	Reps	Tempo	Rest	Weight
❶ Internal/external cable extensions	1	**12-15** each arm, both directions	**311**	**30** secs	
❷ Inverted row	2	**12-15**	**211**	**30** secs	**n/a**
❸ Walking lunge	2	**20**	**212**	**30** secs	**n/a**
❹ Incline press-up	2	**10**	**311**	**30** secs	**n/a**
❺ Gym ball twist crunch	2	**10-12**	**312**	**30** secs	**n/a**
❻ Foot raise and hold	1	**30-60** secs	**n/a**	**n/a**	**n/a**

Warm down and stretch Ten minutes of gentle cardio plus static stretches (20 seconds each). Focus on shoulders, biceps, chest, abs, hams, glutes lower back (see p14)

Notes

❶ Internal/external cable extensions

Target: rotator cuff (internal shoulders)

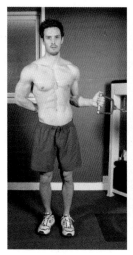 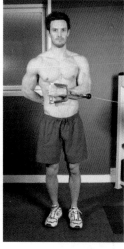 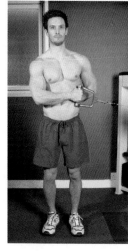 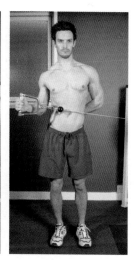

● Stand side-on to a cable set at waist height, grip the handle with your near-side hand.

● While keeping your elbow bent at 90°

and your upper arm by your side, rotate it to bring your hand across your body.

● Grip the handle with the other hand so that your forearm is across your

body, elbow bent at 90° and your upper arm is in line with your body.

● Keeping your upper arm and elbow in position, rotate your arm outwards.

❷ Inverted row

Target: mid-traps, lats, rhomboids

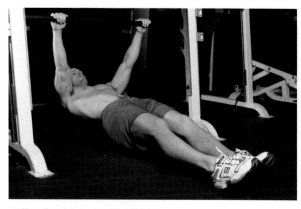 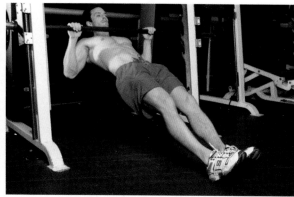

● Hang from a bar set to thigh height, with your heels resting on the ground and your body straight from head to heels.

● Pull your chest up to the bar and squeeze your shoulder blades together, return slowly to the start position.

③ Walking lunge

Target: quads, hamstrings

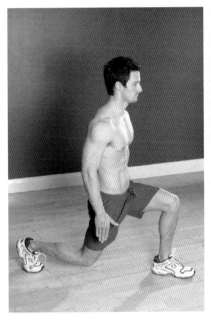
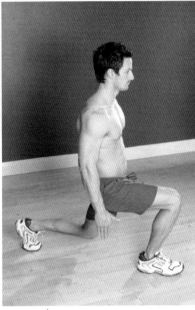

● Stand with your feet apart, keep your back upright and core braced throughout the movement.

● Take a big step forward, keep your front knee over your foot, not beyond it, and lower your back knee until it almost touches the floor.

● Step up, bringing your back leg to meet the front one then repeat the move with the other leg, so that you walk forward with every lunge.

④ Incline press-up

Target: lower pecs, front deltoids, triceps

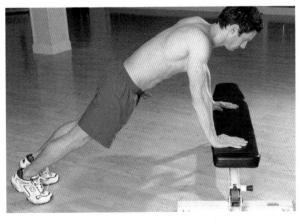
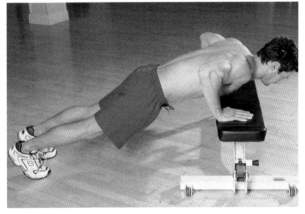

● Place your hands on the bench just wider than shoulder width apart, keep your body straight from shoulders to heels.

● Slowly lower your chest to the bench then press back up powerfully.

⑤ Gym ball twist crunch

Target: abdominals, obliques

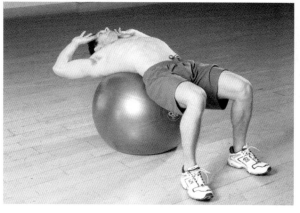 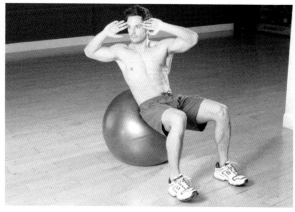

● Touching your fingers to your temples, lean as far back on the ball as you can.

● Keeping your lower back in contact with the ball, contract your abs to curl your chest towards your knees.

● While rising up twist your torso to one side, reverse the movement and repeat on the other side.

⑥ Foot raise and hold

Target: lower abs

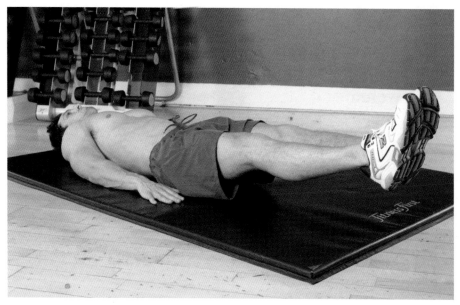

● Lie face up with your hands by your sides and your feet together.

● Brace your core and lift your feet up a few inches while keeping your hips on the floor.

● Hold that position for 30-60 seconds.

WEEK 2
BALANCING ACTS

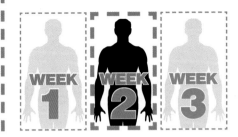

WEEK 1 WEEK 2 WEEK 3

In week two you'll continue to train your stabiliser muscles and core, teaching your body to work as a single unit and getting used to the movements of weight training, without risking injury by doing too much heavy lifting.

You'll also focus on unilateral exercises – moves that work either side of your body independently – so that your stronger side doesn't take all the strain. By training like this, you let your naturally weaker side 'catch up' and ensure that your future muscle gains are balanced.

As you did in week one, concentrate on getting the moves right and controlling the resistance for all the stated reps without compromising good form. And, as in the first week, continue to stick with the light weights for now.

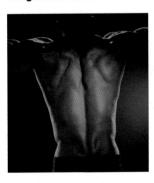

TRAINING PLAN

MON	**WORKOUT A** (see p40)
TUE	**CARDIO SESSION** Run, swim or cycle at RPE level 5 for 20 minutes, maintaining a steady pace
WED	**WORKOUT B** (see p44)
THU	**REST DAY**
FRI	**WORKOUT C** (see p48)
SAT	**CARDIO SESSION** Run, swim or cycle at RPE level 5 for 20 minutes, maintaining a steady pace
SUN	**REST DAY**

MEAL PLAN

Breakfast	Snack
2 boiled eggs with 2 slices wholemeal toast. 250ml pineapple juice.	150g muesli with 150ml whole milk. Add 4 sliced strawberries and a handful of mixed seeds.
150g muesli soaked in 50ml apple juice. Add 30g of dried fruit and 30g of mixed nuts.	Smoothie: blend 250g natural yoghurt, 75g raspberries, 75g blueberries, 100ml apple juice, 1tbsp honey, 1tbsp cold-pressed flax seed oil, 4-6 ice cubes.
100g muesli with 1 chopped mango and 250g natural yoghurt. 1 banana.	115g tuna mixed with 1 chopped tomato and 1 chopped onion on 125g spinach and 75g wholemeal pasta.
3 Shredded Wheat with 300ml skimmed milk and 2tsp raisins. 250ml apple and mango juice.	Protein shake made with 500ml semi-skimmed milk.
4 Weetabix with 250ml skimmed milk, 25g strawberries and a kiwi fruit. 250ml fresh orange juice.	1 apple. 150g low-fat yoghurt mixed with 25g hazelnuts.
4 Weetabix topped with 2 chopped bananas. 140ml orange juice.	150g smoked salmon on wholemeal pitta bread.
Mix 100g porridge oats, 600ml skimmed milk and 40g nuts. 140ml orange juice.	Smoothie: blend 1 scoop protein powder, 2 ice cubes, 220g low-fat natural yoghurt, 60g sliced strawberries and ½ banana with 200ml semi-skimmed milk.

WEEK 4
WEEK 5
WEEK 6
WEEK 7
WEEK 8
WEEK 9
WEEK 10
WEEK 11
WEEK 12

Lunch	Snack	Dinner	Snack	Total
125g sardines on 125g mixed salad (lettuce, cucumber, ½ carrot grated and 1tbsp balsamic vinegar).	1 wholemeal bagel with cream cheese.	Vegetarian curry: boil ½ cup of lentils for 10 minutes. Fry 1 chopped onion and ½ chopped aubergine in olive oil. Add ½tsp turmeric powder, ½tsp cumin, ½tsp curry powder, carton of coconut milk and boiled lentils. Simmer for 15 minutes. Add 125g spinach simmer fo 5 minutes. Serve with 70g wild rice.	5 dried apricots.	**2,916 calories** 212g protein 400g carbs 52g fat
200g grilled chicken cooked in sesame oil with 100g cabbage, 1 sliced carrot, 30g radishes and ginger to flavour.	1 slice of wholemeal toast spread with peanut butter. 3 dried figs.	Vegetarian lasagne using egg pasta sheets, 1 diced courgette, 1 chopped aubergine and 1 tin chopped tomatoes. Layer the vegetables with the pasta sheets. Mix 120ml whole milk, 50g melted butter and 2tbsp wholemeal flour to make a thick sauce and add this to the top layer. Top with a small amount of grated cheese.	1 slice of wholemeal toast spread with peanut butter.	**3,048 calories** 226g protein 410g carbs 56g fat
2 large wholemeal crackers with cream cheese and 1 sliced tomato.	2 wholemeal pitta breads. Celery and carrot sticks with hummus.	200g grilled rump beef steak with braised mangetout, baby carrots, baby sweet corn. Add lime juice and chopped parsley for flavour. 1 grilled pear sprinkled with cinnamon.	30g walnuts.	**3,012 calories** 235g protein 401g carbs 52g fat
1 wholemeal pitta filled with 85g cottage cheese and 50g mixed salad leaves.	1 orange. 2 bananas.	Grill 2 bean burgers and bake a medium-sized sweet potato. Grate 85g carrots and 85g courgettes over the bean burgers and sprinkle with Parmesan to taste.	125g low-fat yoghurt.	**2,530 calories** 145g protein 379g carbs 61g fat
Turkey omelette, made with 3 egg whites, 2 egg yolks and 50g turkey.	Potein shake made with 500ml semi-skimmed milk.	Turkey noodles: grill 1 turkey breast. Chop and mix with 100g cooked noodles. Add soy sauce and lemon juice to taste.	1 chopped apple.	**2,598 calories** 189g protein 422g carbs 52g fat
2 slices of chicken and 50g low fat coleslaw with rocket in 2 seeded rolls.	½ wholemeal bagel topped with 1tbsp raisins, 1tsp peanut butter and 200g cottage cheese. 250ml orange juice.	Spaghetti bolognese with 100g lean minced beef, 100g kidney beans, small tin of chopped tomatoes, 2tbsp tomato purée, diced carrot, 1 crushed garlic clove, ½ chopped red onion, 1tbsp olive oil, dried oregano, fresh basil. Serve with 50g wholemeal spaghetti.	12 almonds.	**2,827 calories** 168g protein 427g carbs 52g fat
Fill a bread roll with 100g roast beef, 220g lettuce, 15g low-fat cheddar, 1 tomato and 2tbsp mustard. 250ml orange juice.	Smoothie: blend 500ml skimmed chocolate milk with 2 bananas, 2tsp whey protein powder and ice cubes.	Teriyaki chicken: mix 75g prepared teriyaki sauce, 75ml orange juice, 1tsp corn starch and ⅓tsp ginger. Stir-fry 115g chicken in ½tbsp olive oil, then remove from pan. Stir-fry 350g broccoli, then add the chicken and sauce and stir. Add 225g water chestnuts. Serve with 50g rice.	Glass of milk.	**2,791 calories,** 177g protein, 372g carbs, 75g fat

WORKOUT A

When you perform unilateral (one-sided) exercises, start with your weaker side. You'll have more energy to target weaker muscles, helping to balance out your strength gains.

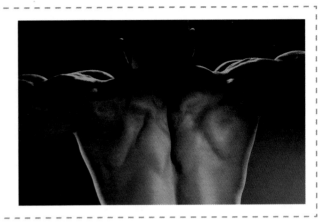

Warm-up Ten minutes of gentle cardio followed by dynamic stretches (see p13)

Exercise		Sets	Reps	Tempo	Rest	Weight
① One-leg squat		2	10-12 each side	311	30 secs	n/a
② Alternating hammer curl with twist		2	14-16	211	30 secs	
③ Alternating dumb-bell shoulder press		2	14-16	211	30 secs	
④ One-leg gym ball curl		2	10 each side	311	30 secs	n/a
⑤ One-arm cable row		2	12-15 each arm	311	30 secs	
⑥ One-arm cable cross crunch		2	12-15 each side	311	30 secs	

Warm down and stretch Ten minutes of gentle cardio plus static stretches (20 seconds each). Focus on quads, hams, glutes shoulders, biceps, abs, upper back (see p14)

Notes

❶ One-leg squat

Target: quads, glutes, hamstrings

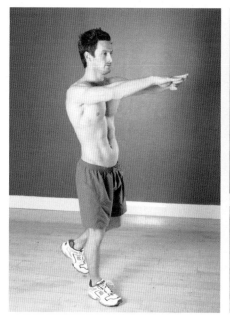
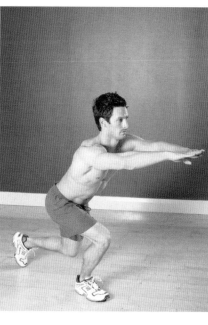

- Stand on one leg with the other slightly off the floor behind you and your hands out in front for balance.
- Keeping your knee in line with your foot and a natural arch in your back, lower yourself until your knee is bent at 90°.

❷ Alternating hammer curl with twist

Target: biceps

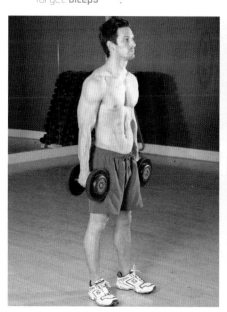
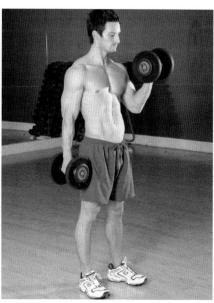

- Hold the dumb-bells by your sides with your palms facing in, keep your back straight, shoulders back and core braced.
- Curl one arm up at a time, keep your upper arms still and don't lean back.
- At the top of the movement twist your palm inwards, reverse and lower under control.

③ Alternating dumb-bell shoulder press

Target: deltoids

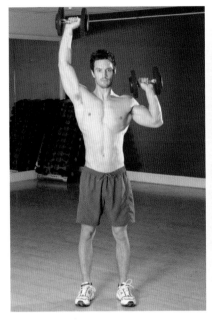 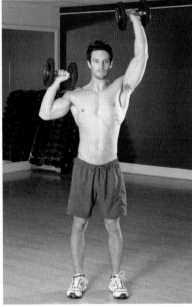

● Stand with your feet shoulder width apart, your torso upright and core braced.

● Start with one dumb-bell raised straight up over your shoulder and the other at shoulder level.

● As you lower one dumb-bell, raise the other, using your core muscles to avoid rocking from side to side.

④ One-leg gym ball curl

Target: hamstrings

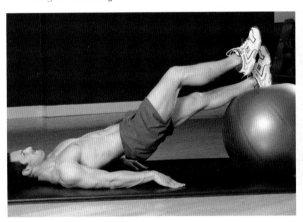 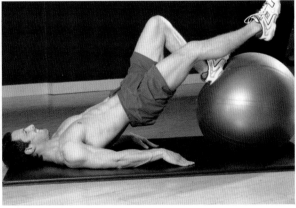

● Rest your head and shoulders on the mat, place one heel on the ball and hold the other slightly raised.

● Keep your body straight from shoulders to heels and your arms by your sides.

● Curl the ball in towards your backside using your heel, keep your hips raised, pause at the top of the movement and return under control.

⑤ One-arm cable row

Target: traps, lats, rhomboids, rear deltoids

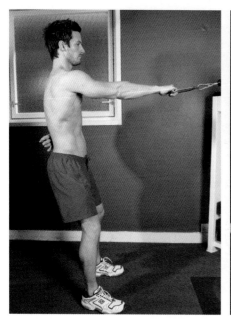 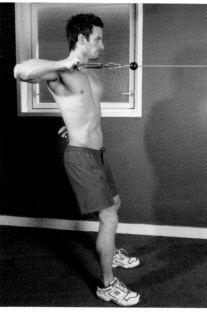

● Stand facing a cable set at shoulder height with your feet shoulder width apart and torso upright.

● Holding your body straight, use one hand to draw the cable back, squeeze at the top of the movement then lower slowly back to the start.

⑥ One-arm cable cross crunch

Target: upper abdominals, obliques

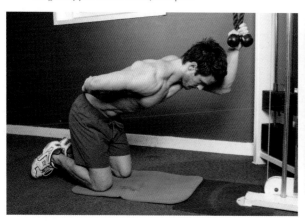 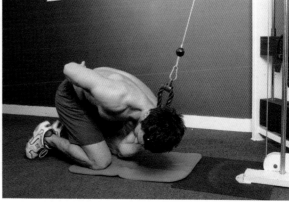

● Hold a high cable in one hand, keep your body straight.

● Using your abs, not your arm, pull the handle down then twist so your elbow touches the opposite knee

WORKOUT B

Some of the moves in this workout are quite complex, so aim to keep your core muscles tight to ensure good posture thoughout.

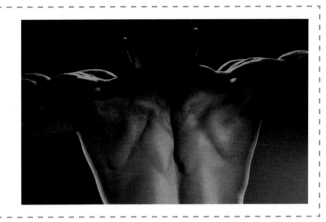

Warm-up Ten minutes of gentle cardio followed by dynamic stretches (see p13)

Exercise		Sets	Reps	Tempo	Rest	Weight
1 Cable lateral lunge		2	**12-15** each side	**311**	**30** secs	
2 Unilateral wall press-up		2	**12-15** each arm	**311**	**30** secs	**n/a**
3 Unilateral lat pull down		2	**12-15** each arm	**311**	**30** secs	
4 Dumb-bell step-up		2	**12-15** each leg	**311**	**30** secs	
5 One-arm one-leg plank		2	**8-10** each side	**222**	**30** secs	**n/a**
6 Front/lateral raise		2	**14-16**	**311**	**30** secs	

Warm down and stretch Ten minutes of gentle cardio plus static stretches (20 seconds each). Focus on adductors, quads, glutes chest, triceps, lats, lower back (see p14)

Notes

① Cable lateral lunge

Target: adductors, quads, hamstrings

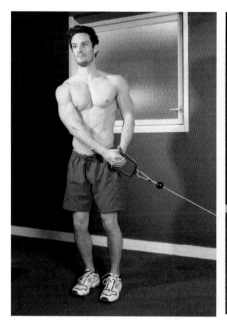 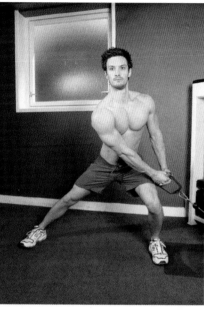

● Stand side-on to a low cable with your torso upright.

● Step sideways towards the cable, lowering onto your leading leg while keeping your knee in line with your foot.

● Stay facing forward, keeping your torso upright and push back up to your starting position.

② Unilateral wall press-up

Target: pecs, triceps

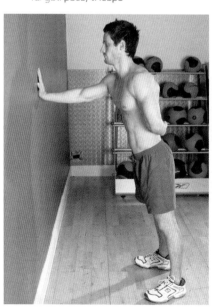 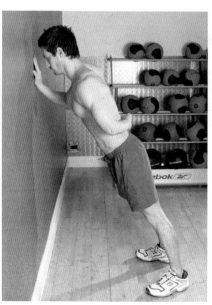

● Stand with your feet slightly wider than shoulder width apart and place one hand on the wall.

● Hold your body in a straight line and lower yourself towards the wall while keeping your elbow close to your side.

③ Unilateral lat pull down

Target: lats, traps, rhomboids, triceps, biceps

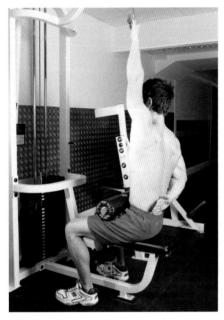 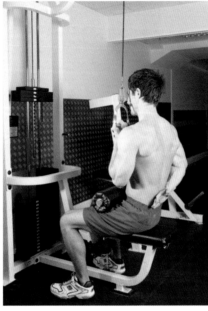

● Adjust the pad so it sits snugly on your thighs. Keep your torso upright and grip the handle with your palm facing away from you.

● Without leaning back pull the cable down to your chest while turning your palm to face you.

④ Dumb-bell step up

Target: quads, glutes

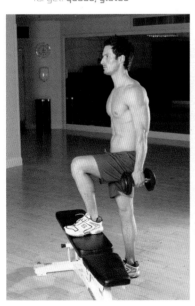 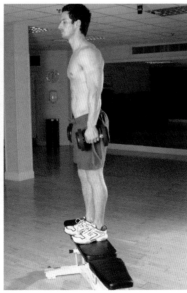

● Using a bench no higher than knee height, keep your back upright and hold the dumb-bells by your side.

● Place one foot on the bench and drive yourself up using the leading leg.

● Step down with the trailing leg and repeat for all reps before swapping legs.

⑤ One arm one leg plank

Target: **core**

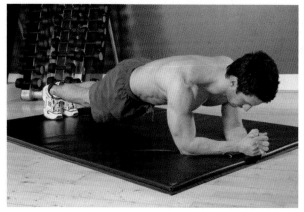 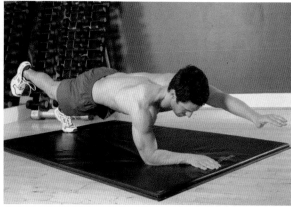

● Position yourself with your feet together and elbows directly beneath your shoulders so that your body is straight from head to heels.

● Keeping your head looking down, lift one leg, and the opposite arm, up and hold out straight.

● Hold this position for a two-count and then repeat with the opposite arm and leg lifted.

⑥ Front/lateral raise

Target: **front and middle deltoids**

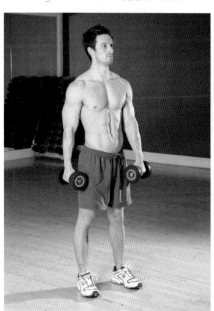 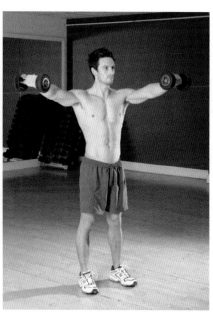

● Stand with your feet shoulder width apart, body upright and core braced.

● Using light dumb-bells hold one by your side and the other in front of you, palms facing in.

● Keeping your arms straight lift to the side and the front simultaneously without swinging your body for momentum.

● Stop lifting at shoulder height and hold for a moment before lowering slowly and alternating sides.

WORKOUT C

This is the last workout of the preliminary stage, so keep concentrating on getting the form right and making every move stable and controlled.

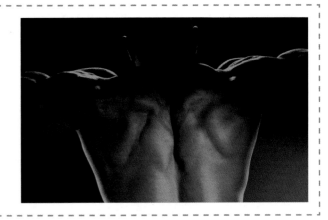

Warm-up Ten minutes of gentle cardio followed by dynamic stretches (see p13)

Exercise		Sets	Reps	Tempo	Rest	Weight
1	Split dumb-bell Romanian deadlift	2	12-15 each side	311	30 secs	
2	Gym ball dumb-bell press	2	12-15	311	30 secs	
3	Side step up	2	12-15 each side	311	30 secs	
4	Diagonal cable raise	2	12-15 each arm	311	30 secs	
5	Lower body Russian twist	2	10	202	30 secs	n/a
6	Split squat to one-arm row	2	12-15 each side	311	30 secs	

Warm down and stretch Ten minutes of gentle cardio plus static stretches (20 seconds each). Focus on hams, glutes, chest, lower back (see p14)

Notes

① Split dumb-bell Romanian deadlift

Target: **hamstrings**

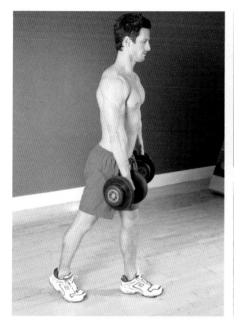 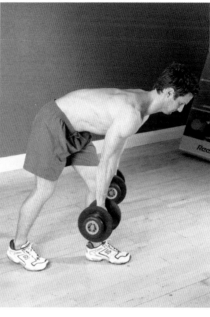

● Start in a split stance with your torso upright, core braced and shoulders back.

● Initiate the movement by leaning forward from the hips, not the waist, bending your knees slightly.

● The weights should travel down alongside your front shin until you feel a good stretch in your hamstrings.

● Ensure your neck is in line with your spine, your back is flat and your core remains braced throughout the movement.

② Gym ball dumb-bell press

Target: **pecs, triceps**

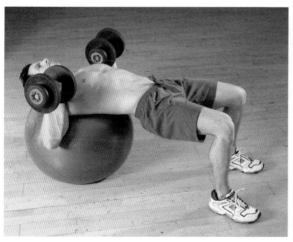 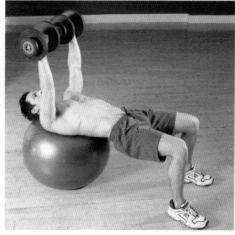

● Support your head and shoulders on the gym ball with your knees bent at 90°.

● Brace your core to keep your body in a straight line from shoulder to knees.

● Hold the dumb-bells at chest height with your palms facing forward, press them up, then slowly lower to the start.

③ Side step up

Target: **glutes, quads, adductors**

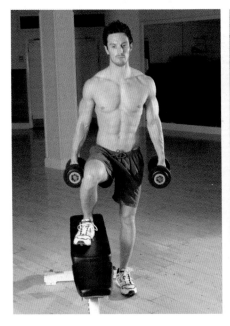 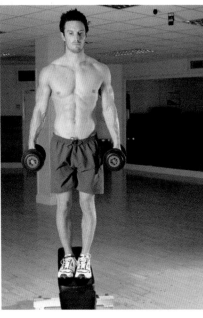

- Using a bench no higher than knee height, keep your back upright and hold the dumb-bells by your side.
- Standing side on to the bench, place one foot on it and drive yourself up using the leading leg.
- Step down to the same side and repeat for all reps before swapping legs.

④ Diagonal cable raise

Target: **deltoids**

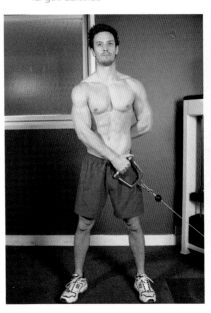 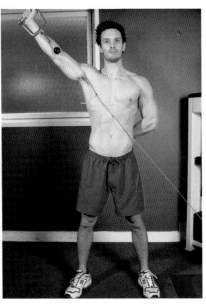

- Stand side-on to a low cable, feet shoulder width apart, torso upright.
- Keeping your core braced and your arm straight, lift the handle across your body.
- Reverse the movement in a slow and controlled manner.

⑤ **Lower body Russian twist**

Target: **lower abdominals**

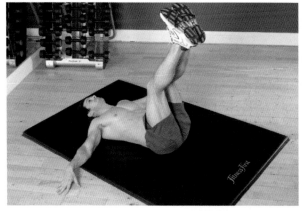 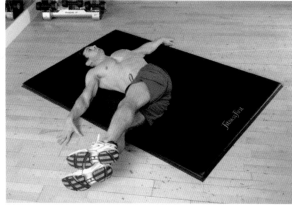

● Lie on your back with your arms out to the sides for balance and your legs straight up in the air.

● Lower your legs to one side, keeping your legs straight and your shoulders flat to the floor.

● Don't let your legs touch the floor, raise your legs back to the start and repeat to the other side.

⑥ **Split squat to one-arm row**

Target: **legs, back, arms, shoulders, core**

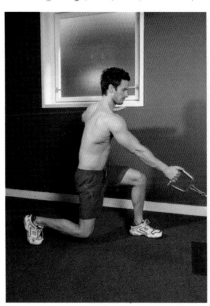 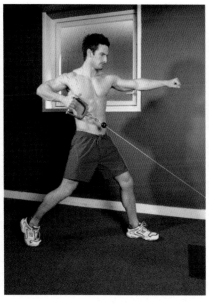

● Start in a lunge position with your left leg forward and your right hand gripping a low cable handle.

● Turn your body towards the cable, keep your head upright and your core braced.

● Without moving your feet, stand up, draw the cable back to your side and retract your shoulder blade while turning your body away from the cable.

WEEK 3

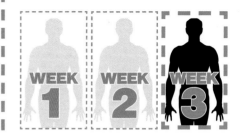

BUILDING ENDURANCE

In the third week you'll focus on muscle endurance. By doing large numbers of reps with relatively light weights you will not only burn a lot of calories from fat, but you will set up new capillary networks in your muscles, providing them with energy that can be used for muscle growth in later weeks when you'll be lifting heavier weights for fewer reps.

You'll also do an interval cardio session. This is when you combine short fast periods of exertion with slower recovery periods. For example, you might sprint for one minute followed by running slowly for two minutes, then repeat the pattern several times. This kind of training has been proven to be effective at burning fat stores and increasing cardiovascular fitness.

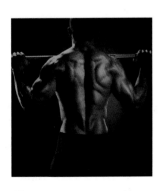

TRAINING PLAN

MON	**WORKOUT A** (see p54)
TUE	**CARDIO SESSION** 20-minute running intervals 4 minutes warm-up – level 2 1 minute fast – level 8 2 minutes slow – level 4 } x3 4 minutes warm down – level 2
WED	**WORKOUT B** (see p58)
THU	**REST DAY**
FRI	**WORKOUT C** (see p62)
SAT	**CARDIO SESSION** Recovery Run, swim or cycle at level 5 for 30 minutes, maintaining a steady pace
SUN	**REST DAY**

MEAL PLAN

Breakfast	Snack
120g oats, 75g bran, 3 strawberries, 1 sliced banana and ½ scoop of whey protein mixed with water.	Raisin, cranberry and almond snack bar.
French toast: 2 whole eggs, 3 slices wholemeal bread, 110ml milk and ½tsp cinnamon. Serve with 6tbsp cottage cheese and small tin sliced peaches.	Raisin, cranberry and almond snack bar.
2 slices of wholemeal toast. 125g low-fat yoghurt with 30g honey.	Whey protein shake made with 500ml semi-skimmed milk.
2 bananas, 30g honey and 50g peanut butter on 2 slices wholemeal toast.	Smoothie: blend 500ml skimmed milk, 2 bananas and 2 scoops whey protein.
Omelette made with 4 egg whites and 2 yolks. 1 plain bagel.	250g live yoghurt with 100g dried pineapple.
2 eggs scrambled with 50ml whole milk on 1 slice wholemeal toast. 250ml pineapple juice.	100g chicken with hummus.
50g granola with 350g low-fat plain yoghurt, 200g chopped strawberries, 1tbsp brown sugar and 1 scoop protein powder.	Blend 1½ bananas and 2 scoops protein powder with 500ml of water.

| WEEK 4 | WEEK 5 | WEEK 6 | WEEK 7 | WEEK 8 | WEEK 9 | WEEK 10 | WEEK 11 | WEEK 12 |

Lunch	Snack	Dinner	Snack	Total
Salmon sandwich: 110g tinned salmon, 2tbsp light mayonnaise, 1tsp horseradish, 2 finely chopped spring onions and a pinch of parsley on 4 slices wholemeal bread.	250g low-fat yoghurt with 1tbsp toasted chopped pecan nuts.	Grill 115g skinless chicken breasts, in 2tsp of lemon and herb seasoning, for 7-10 minutes each side. Peel and slice 2 large potatoes, then put in a plastic bag and add a dash of ground pepper, 2tsp extra virgin olive oil and ¼tsp rosemary. Toss the bag so the potatoes are coated and roast for 20-30 minutes.	75g pineapple.	**2,823 calories** 114g protein 440g carbs 70g fat
Turkey omelette: 4 large eggs, 2 small onions, 85g cooked turkey, handful of kidney beans, 1 chopped green pepper, handful of chopped mushrooms and black pepper.	2 slices wholemeal toast with 25g peanut butter and 1 chopped banana.	Bake 2 potatoes and fill with 1tsp of margarine and salt and pepper. Pan-fry 115g of lean sirloin steak for 5-10 minutes and sauté 30g mushrooms in 1tsp olive oil. Serve the mushrooms on the steak.	1 slice wholemeal toast with 25g peanut butter. Glass of milk.	**2,850 calories** 160g protein 362g carbs 78g fat
500g mixed sushi pack.	150g mixed fruit salad (kiwi fruit, raspberries, apples and grapes).	Salsa chicken and pasta: cook 1 chicken breast, 85g wholemeal pasta, 125g broccoli and 125g carrots. Chop and mix with 30g salsa and a dash of Tabasco.	Cereal bar.	**2,550 calories** 191g protein 350g carbs 54g fat
Fill 2 bagels with cottage cheese. 50g pineapple.	Raisin, cranberry and almond snack bar.	Grill a 200g salmon fillet for 6-8 minutes each side and serve with 85g brown rice and 125g spinach.	Pot of low-fat yoghurt topped with 1tsp of mixed seeds.	**2,790 calories** 158g protein 393g carbs 66g fat
Fill 2 wholemeal sub rolls with 50g chicken and salad leaves. 1 small smoothie.	Whey protein shake made with 500ml semi-skimmed milk.	Grill a chicken breast for 15 minutes. Place a clove of crushed garlic and ½ chopped onion in a pan and cook for 5 minutes until browned. Add the chicken and 200g tinned tomatoes, with chilli powder or sliced green chillies to taste. Cover and cook for a further 5-10 minutes. Serve with 75g brown rice	Glass of skimmed milk.	**2,624 calories** 159g protein 393g carbs 41g fat
2 granary bagels with goat's cheese, sun-blanched tomatoes and 1 handful of flax seeds.	125g strawberries and 2-3 dried prunes with 250g natural yoghurt.	Stir-fry 150g duck with 1 chopped onion, 1 chopped courgette and 50g mushrooms. Serve with 75g quinoa.	1 kiwi fruit and 1 plum.	**2,942 calories** 228g protein 395g carbs 50g fat
½ wholemeal bagel topped with 1tbsp raisins, 1tsp peanut butter and 200g cottage cheese. 250ml orange juice.	250g low-fat yoghurt with 75g pineapple.	2 chicken fajitas made with a chopped grilled chicken breast, 15g sliced mushrooms, ½ sliced onion, 1 red pepper and 30g low-fat cheese.	12 almonds.	**2,839 calories** 165g protein 472g carbs 55g fat

WORKOUT A

You're working on muscle endurance in this phase of the plan, so you'll do three sets of most exercises while keeping the rep rate high. Pick a weight that allows you to complete all your reps before failure.

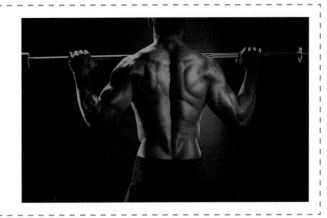

Warm-up Ten minutes of gentle cardio followed by dynamic stretches (see p13)

Exercise		Sets	Reps	Tempo	Rest	Weight
1 Squat to curl to press		3	15-20	311	45 secs	
2 Lat pull down		3	15-20	311	45 secs	
3 Triceps press down		3	15-20	311	45 secs	
4 Crunch		3	15-20	311	45 secs	n/a
5 Gym ball leg curl		3	10-15	311	45 secs	n/a
6 Gym ball back extension		3	10-15	311	45 secs	n/a

Warm down and stretch Ten minutes of gentle cardio plus static stretches (20 seconds each). Focus on quads, hams, glutes, back, abs, triceps (see p14)

Notes

① Squat to curl to press

Target: legs, arms, shoulders

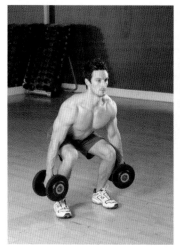 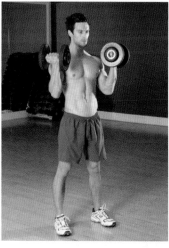 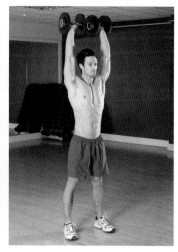

● Start in a squat position with a natural arch in your back, and your knees in line with your feet.

● Drive up through your heels and curl the dumb-bells up to your shoulder keeping your elbows by your sides.

● Drive the weights directly overhead, twisting your hands so your palms face outwards.

● Reverse the movement to the start in a controlled manner.

② Lat pull down

Target: lats, traps, rhomboids

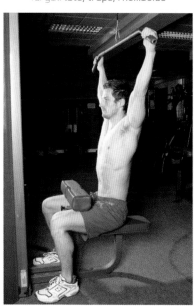 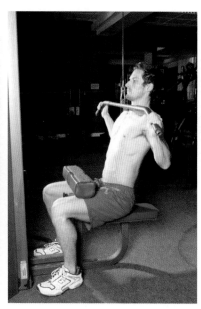

● With your thighs secured snugly under the pad, keep your torso upright and take a wide grip on the bar.

● Without leaning back too far, pull the bar down to your upper chest, and squeeze your lats.

● Allow the bar to raise up to the start, slowly and under control.

③ Triceps press down

Target: triceps

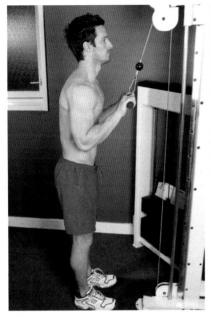
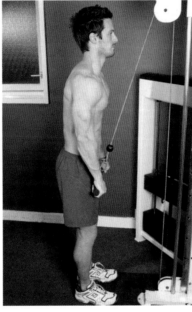

● Stand in front of a cable set at head height. If it helps your balance then place one foot in front of the other.

● Without leaning forward press the bar down and squeeze your triceps at the bottom of the move.

● Keep your back straight and your elbows tucked in throughout the movement.

④ Crunch

Target: upper abdominals

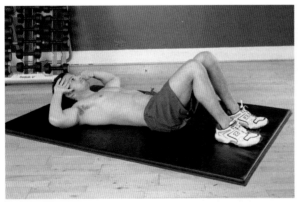

● Lie with your feet flat on the floor, knees bent at 90° and your head off the mat.

● Touch your fingers to your temples to avoid pulling on your neck.

● Keeping your lower back in contact with the mat, contract your abs to lift your shoulders off the mat, curling your chest towards your knees.

● Pause at the top of the move, squeeze your abs and lower slowly to the start.

⑤ Gym ball leg curl

Target: hamstrings

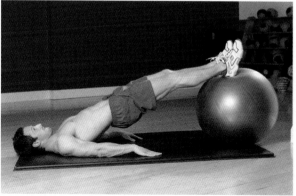 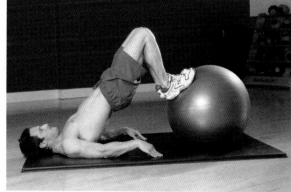

● Rest your head and shoulders on the floor and your heels on top of the ball, your body should be straight from shoulders to heels.

● Raise your hips and drag the ball towards your backside with your heels, keeping your body straight.

● Pause at the top of the movement and return slowly to the start.

⑥ Gym ball back extension

Target: lower back

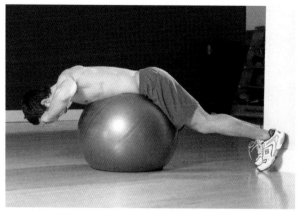 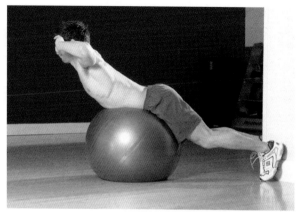

● Wrap your body around the gym ball, jamming your feet against a wall for support.

● Lift your back until your body forms a straight line, being careful not to over-extend.

● Pause for a moment at the top of the exercise before lowering slowly.

WORKOUT B

Keep the weights light but the work rate high as you continue to develop your muscle endurance with this workout.

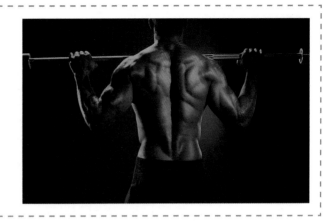

Warm up Ten minutes of gentle cardio followed by dynamic stretches (see p13)

Exercise		Sets	Reps	Tempo	Rest	Weight
1 Lunge to press		3	16-20	211	45 secs	
2 Upright row		3	15-20	311	45 secs	
3 Incline dumb-bell curl		3	15-20	311	45 secs	
4 Dumb-bell gym ball squat		3	15-20	311	45 secs	
5 Gym ball dumb-bell pullover		3	15-20	311	45 secs	
6 Bicycles		3	20 secs	101	45 secs	n/a

Warm down and stretch Ten minutes of gentle cardio plus static stretches (20 seconds each). Focus on quads, hams, glutes, biceps, chest, abs (see p14)

Notes

❶ Lunge to press

Target: quads, glutes, hamstrings, deltoids, triceps

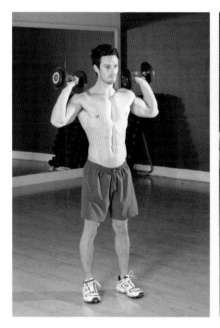
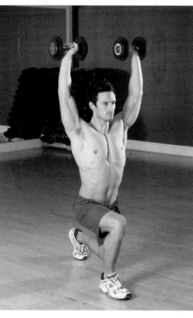

- Stand with your back straight and your core braced, holding the dumb-bells at shoulder height.

- Step forward into a lunge, keeping your front knee over your foot and bringing your back knee close to the ground.

- Simultaneously press the weights directly overhead while maintaining a natural arch in your spine.

- Reverse the movement to return to the start, and alternate legs with each rep.

❷ Upright row

Target: upper traps, deltoids

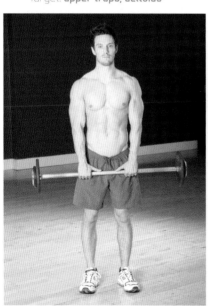
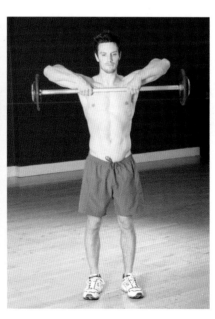

- Stand upright with your shoulders back, gripping the bar in front of your thighs.

- Brace your core and draw the weight up, raising your elbows high to the sides.

- Pause for a moment at the top of the movement before slowly lowering.

③ Incline dumb-bell curl

Target: **biceps**

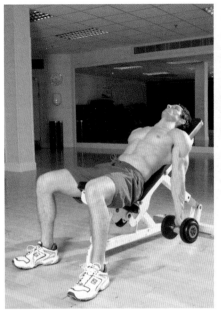
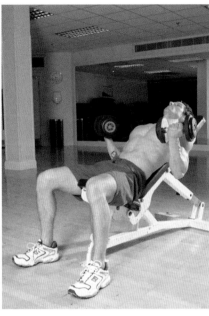

● Sit on a bench set at 30-45° with your feet flat on the floor and your back against the pad.

● Let your arms hang straight down with your palms facing forward.

● Without lifting your head or back, curl the dumb-bells up, turning your wrists slightly outwards at the top.

④ Dumb-bell gym ball squat

Target: **quads, glutes, core**

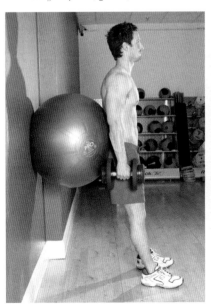
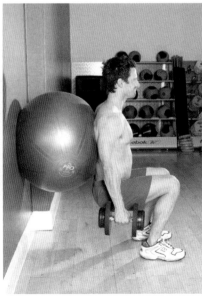

● Stand with feet shoulder width apart, core braced and the ball behind your lower back.

● Lower into the squat until your thighs are parallel with the floor, allowing the ball to roll up your back as you move.

● Drive up to reverse the movement, rolling the ball as you do.

⑤ Gym ball dumb-bell pullover

Target: pecs, lats, core

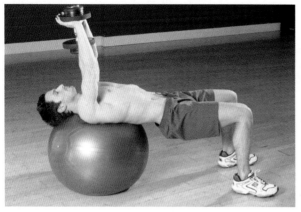 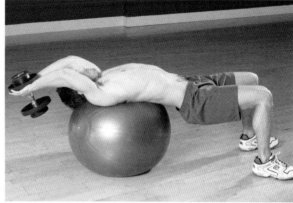

● Support your head and shoulders on the ball with a dumb-bell in both hands over your chest.

● Your feet should be flat on the ground, your core engaged and your body straight from head to knees.

● Keeping a slight bend in your elbows, slowly lower the weight behind your head.

● Pull the weight back to the start using your chest muscles. Avoid arching your back to aid the movement.

⑥ Bicycles

Target: abdominals

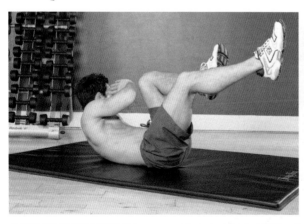

● Start with your fingers by your temples, crunch up to bring your right elbow to your left knee while extending your right leg.

● Twist your torso to the other side as you crunch your left elbow to your right knee and extend your left leg.

● Perform this movement in a quick but controlled manner, being careful not to strain your neck.

WORKOUT C

Concentrate on keeping your core engaged throughout each set to ensure you maintain a good posture.

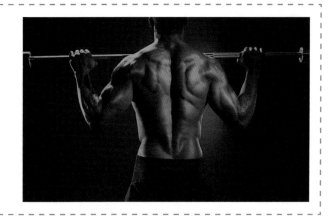

Warm-up Ten minutes of gentle cardio followed by dynamic stretches (see p13)

Exercise		Sets	Reps	Tempo	Rest	Weight
1 Rotating squat press		3	16-20	311	45 secs	
2 Wide-grip cable row		3	15-20	311	45 secs	
3 Dumb-bell bench press		3	15-20	311	45 secs	
4 Dumb-bell lateral lunge and touch		3	8-10 each side	211	45 secs	
5 Seated reverse crunch		3	10-15	311	45 secs	n/a
6 Supine gym ball calf raise		3	15-20	211	45 secs	n/a

Warm down and stretch Ten minutes of gentle cardio plus static stretches (20 seconds each). Focus on quads, hams, glutes, adductors, chest, triceps, abs, calves (see p14)

Notes

❶ Rotating squat press

Target: legs, back, shoulder, arms, core

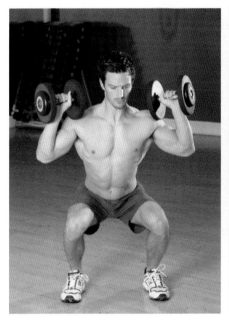 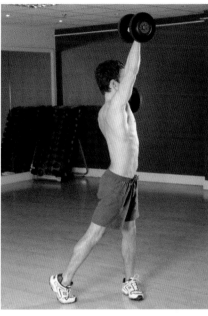

● With the dumb-bells at shoulder level drop into a squat, maintaining a natural arch in your back.

● As you drive up, rotate your body and press one dumb-bell overhead, lifting your heel as you turn.

● Return to the start and repeat the move on the other side.

❷ Wide-grip cable row

Target: mid traps, lats, rhomboids, rear deltoids

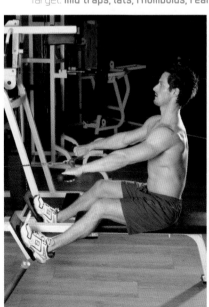 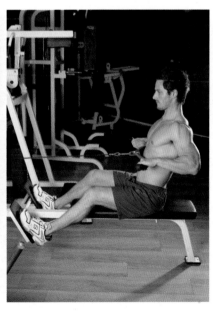

● Sit with a slight bend in your knees, your back straight and your shoulder blades retracted.

● Take a wide grip on the bar and ensure that there is tension in the cable.

● Keeping upper body movement to a minimum, pull the bar into your sternum and squeeze your shoulder blades together.

③ Dumb-bell bench press

Target: **pecs, triceps**

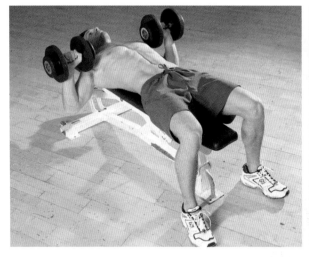 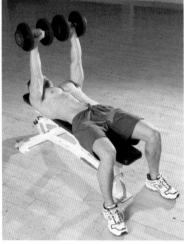

● Lie on a bench with your knees bent at 90° and your feet flat on the ground, holding dumb-bells at chest level.

● Brace your core muscles and without arching your back, press the weights straight up, then slowly lower.

④ Dumb-bell lateral lunge and touch

Target: **hamstrings, adductors**

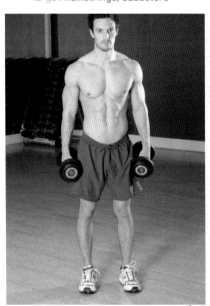 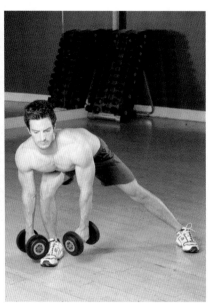

● Stand with your feet close together and your torso upright holding dumb-bells by your sides.

● Take a big step to the side, keep your feet pointing forward and lower onto your leading leg.

● Lean forward from the hips rather than the waist, keep your back flat and lower the weights down your leading leg.

⑤ Seated reverse crunch

Target: **lower abdominals**

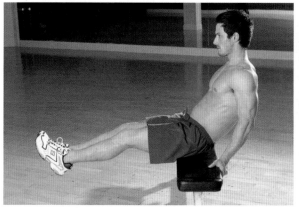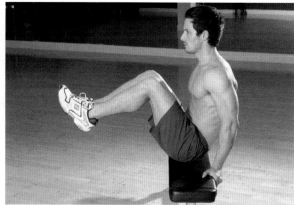

● Sit on the edge of a bench, lean your torso back to around 45° and grip the edge for support.

● Raise your feet out in front then draw your knees into your chest, maintain balance throughout.

⑥ Supine gym ball calf raise

Target: **calves**

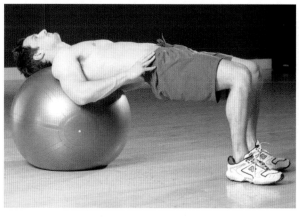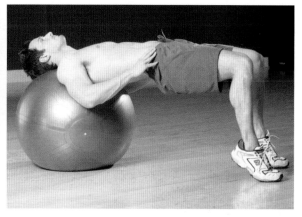

● Rest your head and shoulders on the ball with your knees bent at 90° and your body in a straight line from head to knees.

● Push up onto your toes and hold for a count of two before lowering.

WEEK 4

COMPOUND MOVES

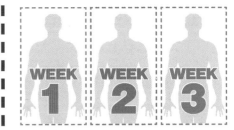

WEEK **1** | WEEK **2** | WEEK **3**

In week four you'll stick with relatively high reps and low weights while you establish the base upon which your muscle training will be built. However, you're going to get an introduction to some of the classic compound moves that will become the staples of your future workouts.

Compound exercises are ones that use several muscle groups at once, releasing waves of natural growth hormone, so they stimulate the most muscle growth. For example, a squat uses muscles in your quads, hamstrings, glutes, core and back.

By using light weights you can focus on getting the form spot on. But this won't make for an easy workout – you'll still be doing 15 to 20 reps per set, and three sets per exercise.

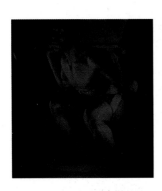

TRAINING PLAN

MON
WORKOUT A
(see p68)

TUE
CARDIO SESSION
20-minute running intervals
4 minutes warm-up – level 2
1 minute fast – level 8 }
2 minutes slow – level 4 } x4
4 minutes warm down – level 2

WED
WORKOUT B
(see p72)

THU
REST DAY

FRI
WORKOUT C
(see p76)

SAT
CARDIO SESSION
Recovery
Run, swim or cycle at level 5 for 30 minutes, maintaining a steady pace

SUN
REST DAY

MEAL PLAN

Breakfast	Snack
Porridge made with 45g oats, 300ml skimmed milk, 1tsp honey and 25g whey protein.	1 mashed banana on 1 slice wholemeal toast.
Smoothie: blend 25g whey protein, 100g strawberries and ½ banana with 300ml skimmed milk and 1tsp flaxseed oil. Serve chilled.	90g sardines on 2 slices wholemeal toast.
Porridge made with 45g oats, 300ml skimmed milk, 1tsp honey and 25g whey protein.	1 apple with 2tbsp peanut butter. Glass of skimmed milk.
Blend 1 mango, 80g blueberries, 2tbsp natural yoghurt, 1tbsp oats and 25g whey protein with 100ml apple juice and 100ml water.	90g sardines on 2 slices wholemeal toast.
4 scrambled egg whites on 2 slices of wholemeal toast. Glass of orange juice.	Mixed nuts, raisins and dried cranberries.
Porridge made with 45g oats, 300ml skimmed milk, 1tsp honey, handful of blueberries and 25g whey protein.	1 mashed banana with 2tbsp peanut butter on 2 slices of wholemeal toast
2 scrambled eggs on 2 slices of wholemeal toast. Glass of orange juice.	30g brazil nuts. Glass of skimmed milk.

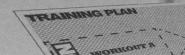

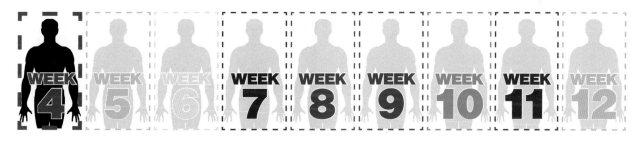

Lunch	Snack	Dinner	Snack	Total
Turkey-salad sandwich on wholemeal bread. 1 apple.	Mixed nuts, raisins and dried cranberries with cottage cheese.	90g wholemeal pasta and 200g grilled chicken with jar of tomato sauce and chopped onion.	Smoothie: blend 25g protein, 50g blueberries, 50g blackberries and ½ banana with 300ml skimmed milk.	**2,865 calories** 205g protein 363g carbs 64g fat
Medium-sized jacket potato with baked beans and cottage cheese.	140g grilled chicken, with beetroot.	200g chicken and vegetable stir-fry with red and green peppers, sesame oil and seeds. 70g brown rice.	Smoothie: blend 25g whey protein, 80g raspberries, 80g blueberries and 50g blackberries, with 200-300ml water.	**2,869 calories** 208g protein 351g carbs 63g fat
Medium-sized jacket potato with tuna, baked beans and grated cheese.	Smoothie: blend 25g whey protein, 80g raspberries, 80g blueberries and 50g blackberries with 200-300ml water.	200g salmon with 175g new potatoes, 70g carrots, courgettes and broccoli.	120g low-fat yoghurt with strawberries.	**2,876 calories** 259g protein 241g carbs 77g fat
Medium-sized jacket potato with baked beans and cottage cheese.	140g grilled chicken with beetroot.	120g tuna steak with stir-fried broccoli, green beans and spinach with sesame oil and seeds. 70g brown rice.	Smoothie: blend 25g whey protein, 80g raspberries, 80g blueberries and 50g blackberries with 250ml water.	**2,910 calories** 212g protein 361g carbs 63g fat
Turkey and cheese bagel. 1 orange.	Blend 25g whey protein, 3 almonds, 3 brazil nuts, 80g blueberries, 2 dates, 50g natural yoghurt and ½ banana with 250ml skimmed milk.	140g lemon sole with stir-fried broccoli, green beans, red peppers and spinach with sesame oil and seeds. 70g brown rice.	Smoothie: blend 25g whey protein, 50g blueberries, 50g blackberries, ½ banana with 300ml skimmed milk.	**2,887 calories** 199g protein 345g carbs 70g fat
Turkey, cheese and mustard bagel. 1 apple.	1 tin of tuna with beetroot and cottage cheese.	120g fillet steak with mashed potato and spinach. Fruit sorbet.	Smoothie: blend 25g whey protein, 80g raspberries, 80g blueberries and 50g blackberries with 250ml water	**2,950 calories** 208g protein 359g carbs 68g fat
Large jacket potato with baked beans, tuna and grated cheese.	Smoothie: blend 25g whey protein, 100g strawberries and ½ banana with 300ml skimmed milk and 1tsp flaxseed oil.	150g roast beef with 100g new potatoes, and mixed vegetables.	100g cottage cheese. 1 apple.	**3,012 calories** 208g protein 367g carbs 73g fat

WORKOUT A

This workout includes some of the classic compound moves you need to learn to add muscle mass. However, at this stage keep the weights light so you can practise the form and continue to build muscle endurance.

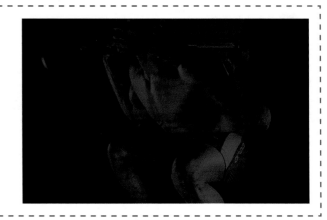

Warm-up Ten minutes of gentle cardio followed by dynamic stretches (see p13)

Exercise		Sets	Reps	Tempo	Rest	Weight
❶ Bench press		3	15-20	311	45 secs	
❷ Bent-over row		3	15-20	311	45 secs	
❸ Squat		3	15-20	311	45 secs	
❹ Shrug		3	15-20	311	45 secs	
❺ Crossover crunch		2	15 each side	311	45 secs	n/a
❻ Gym ball back extension		3	15	311	45 secs	n/a

Warm down and stretch Ten minutes of gentle cardio plus static stretches (20 seconds each). Focus on quads, hams, glutes, chest, triceps, traps, abs (see p14)

Notes

❶ Bench press

Target: **pecs, triceps**

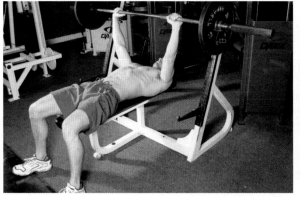

● Lie on the bench with your knees bent at 90°, your feet flat on the floor and your core braced.

● Grip the bar wider than shoulder width, retract your shoulder blades and lift the bar off the rack, holding it directly over your chest.

● Maintain a natural arch in your back. There should just be enough room to slip a few fingers between your lower back and the bench.

● Lower the bar to your chest slowly and press up powerfully.

❷ Bent-over row

Target: **traps, lats, rhomboids**

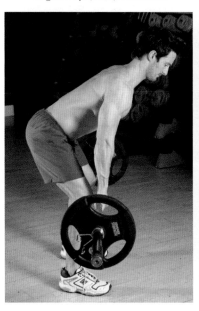 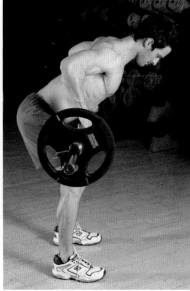

● Start with your core braced, your back straight and your shoulder blades retracted.

● With your knees slightly bent, lean forward from the hips, rather than the waist.

● Grip the bar just wider than shoulder width apart, letting it hang straight down around knee level.

● Pull the bar up into your sternum, squeezing your shoulder blades together at the top of the move, then lower the bar slowly to the start.

③ Squat

Target: quads, glutes, hamstrings

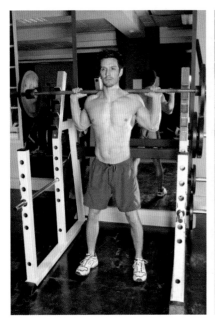
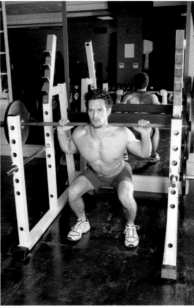

- Stand with your feet shoulder width apart, your toes turned out slightly and your core braced.
- Rest the bar on the back of your shoulders, not your neck, gripping it close to your shoulders.
- Maintain a natural arch in your back, keep your elbows retracted and look forward throughout the movement.
- Lower until your thighs are parallel to the floor, keeping your knees in line with your feet, then push back up through your heels.

④ Shrug

Target: upper traps

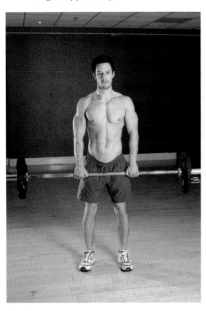
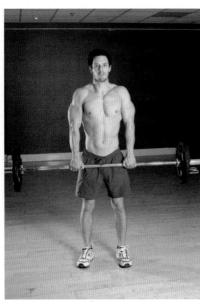

- Stand upright with your shoulders back, grip the bar just outside your thighs.
- Without letting your elbows bend, raise your shoulders straight up and hold for 1-2 seconds.

⑤ Crossover crunch

Target: **abdominals**

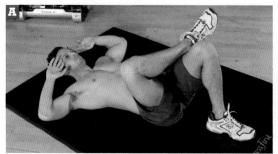

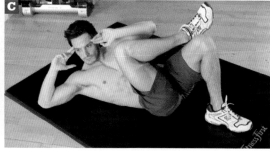

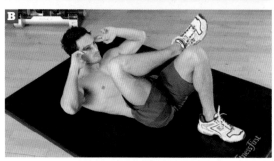

● Lie with your head held off the floor, your fingers touching your temples and your foot resting on the opposite knee.

● Without pulling on your neck contract your abs to lift your shoulders off the floor.

● Twist your torso so your elbow moves to meet your knee, reverse the move slowly back to the start.

⑥ Gym ball back extension

Target: **lower back**

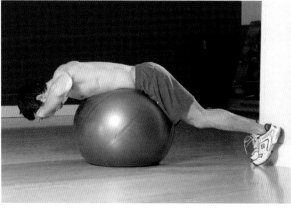

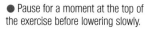

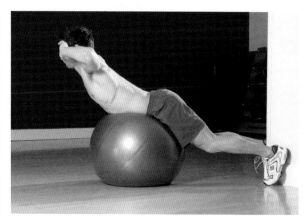

● Wrap your body around the gym ball, jamming your feet against a wall for support.

● Lift your back until your body forms a straight line. Be careful not to over-extend.

● Pause for a moment at the top of the exercise before lowering slowly.

WORKOUT B

You're continuing with the muscle endurance phase in this week. High reps means you'll need to keep the weight manageable. If you find your form wavering towards the end of a set, go lighter for the next set.

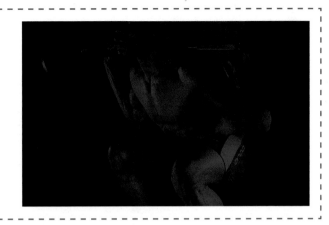

Warm-up Ten minutes of gentle cardio followed by dynamic stretches (see p13)

Exercise		Sets	Reps	Tempo	Rest	Weight
❶ Deadlift		3	15-20	311	45 secs	
❷ Gym ball decline press-up		3	10	311	45 secs	n/a
❸ Negative pull-ups		3	10	5--	45 secs	n/a
❹ Shoulder press		3	15-20	311	45 secs	
❺ Lying triceps extension		3	15-20	311	45 secs	
❻ Plank		1	60 secs	n/a	n/a	n/a

Warm down and stretch Ten minutes of gentle cardio plus static stretches (20 seconds each). Focus on hams, glutes, chest, triceps, lats, shoulders, abs (see p14)

Notes

❶ Deadlift

Target: quads, glutes, hamstrings, back, core

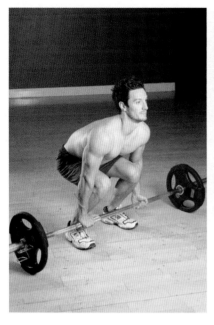 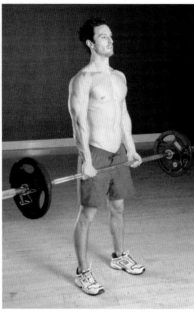

● Start with your feet shoulder width apart, grasp the bar outside your knees with an overhand or alternate grip.

● Position the bar close to your shins with your shoulders directly over it and keep looking forward.

● Ensure you keep your back flat, your shoulders retracted and your core braced.

● Start the lift by pushing with your glutes and pushing down through the heels.

● Keeping your shoulders back, the bar should rise up your shins, as it passes your knees, push your hips forward.

❷ Gym ball decline press-up

Target: pecs, shoulders, triceps, core

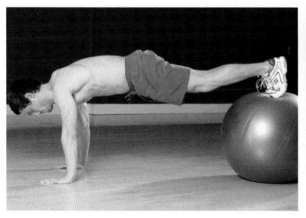 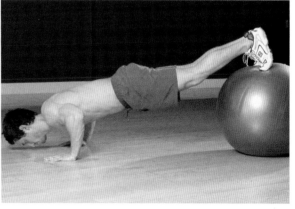

● Start with your hands on the floor beneath your shoulders and your feet together on top of the ball.

● Perform a press-up without letting your hips sag, control any wobble from the ball.

③ Negative pull-ups

Target: lats, traps, rhomboids

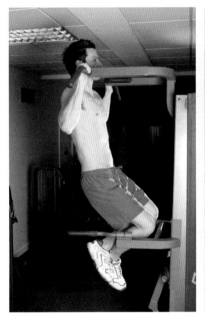
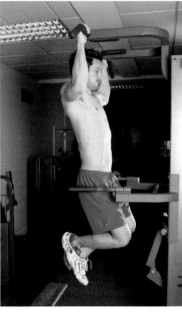

● Grip the bar with an overhand grip just wider than shoulder width apart.

● Use a bench or a helper to get your chin over the bar.

● Lower yourself in a slow and controlled manner until your arms are straight.

④ Shoulder press

Target: deltoids

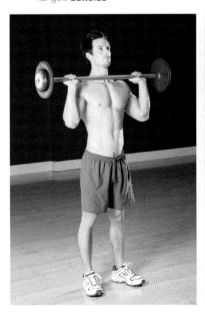
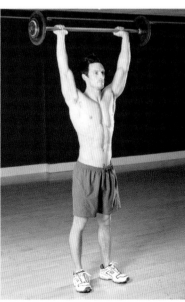

● Stand with your feet shoulder width apart, your body upright, core braced and head looking straight ahead.

● Grip the bar just wider than shoulder width apart and hold it on your upper chest.

● Press the bar directly overhead without tilting your hips forward, slowly lower it to the start.

⑤ Lying triceps extension

Target: **tricep**

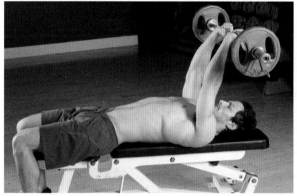 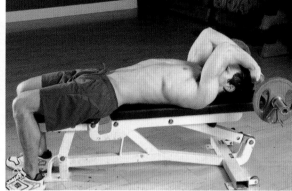

● Lie on a bench with your core braced, knees bent at 90° and feet flat on the ground.

● Hold the EZ-bar over your head, not your chest, with an overhand grip, wrists turned in slightly.

● Without arching your back

lower the bar slowly behind your head while keeping your upper arms angled slightly back.

● Reverse the motion to press the bar back up, squeezing your triceps at the top of the move.

⑥ Plank

Target: **core**

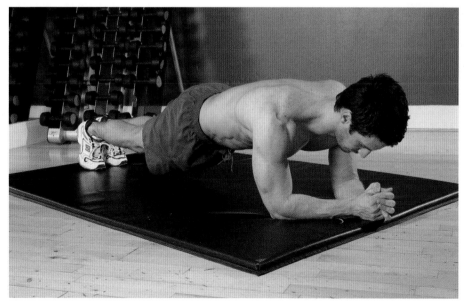

● Position yourself with your feet together and elbows directly beneath your shoulders so that your body is straight from head to heels.

● Keeping your head looking down, hold that position for 60 seconds without letting your hips sag.

WORKOUT C

This is the final endurance workout, so focus on getting to the end of each set with the last rep being as good as the first.

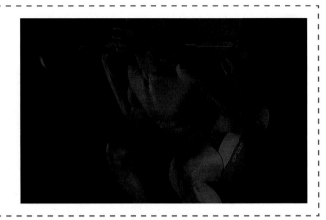

Warm-up Ten minutes of gentle cardio followed by dynamic stretches (see p13)

Exercise		Sets	Reps	Tempo	Rest	Weight
1 Bench dip		3	10-12	311	45 secs	n/a
2 Split squat		3	12 each leg	311	45 secs	
3 EZ-bar curl		3	15-20	311	45 secs	
4 Romanian deadlift		3	15-20	311	45 secs	
5 One-arm reverse flye		3	15-20 each arm	311	45 secs	
6 Bench leg raise		3	10	411	45 secs	n/a

Warm down and stretch Ten minutes of gentle cardio plus static stretches (20 seconds each). Focus on quads, glutes, hams, biceps, back, abs (see p14)

Notes

❶ Bench dip

Target: **triceps**

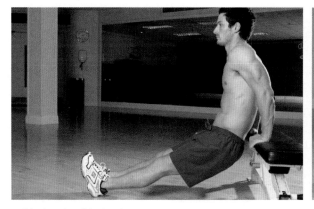 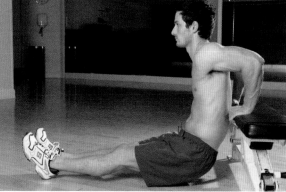

● Grip the edge of the bench with your palms facing back, keep your back upright, legs straight and feet together.

● Lower your body straight down, keeping your elbows pointing back, then press back up powerfully.

❷ Split squat

Target: **quads, glutes, hamstrings**

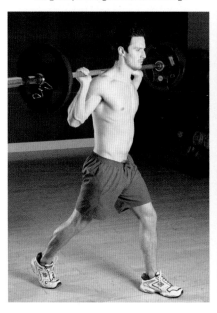 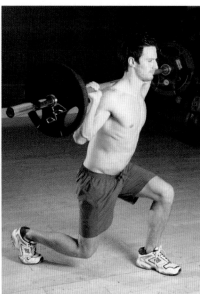

● Start in a split stance with both feet facing forward, back upright and core braced.

● Rest the bar on the back of your shoulders and keep your elbows back to retract your shoulder blades.

● Sink down until your back knee almost touches the floor and your front knee bends to 90°.

❸ EZ-bar curl

Target: biceps

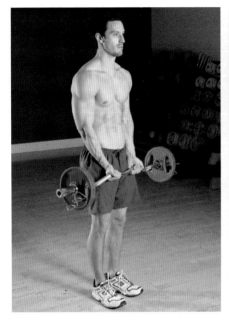
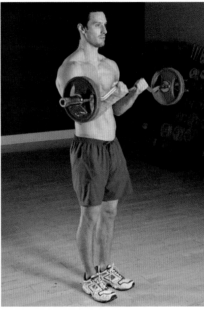

● Stand tall with your shoulders back and your core muscles braced for support.

● Keep your elbows tucked into your sides and grip the EZ-bar with your hands turned inwards slightly.

● Lift the bar without rocking back and forth for momentum, stop before your forearms are vertical and lower slowly.

❹ Romanian deadlift

Target: hamstrings

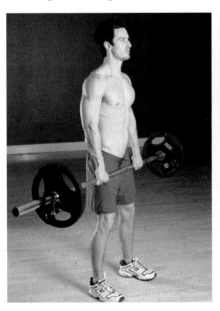
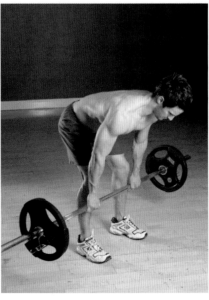

● Stand with your feet shoulder width apart, your head up, looking forward, shoulders back and core braced.

● Grip the bar just outside your hips and initiate the move by leaning forward from the hips rather than the waist.

● Allow a slight bend in your knees, keep your back straight and push your hips back as the bar travels down your shins.

● Lower the bar until you feel a good stretch in your hamstrings then reverse the movement to the start.

⑤ One-arm reverse flye

Target: **traps, rear deltoids**

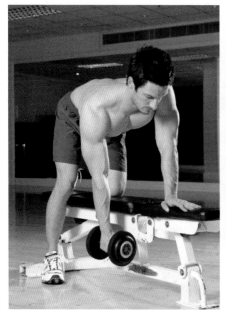
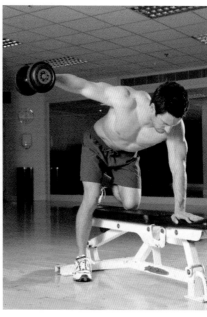

● Start with one hand and knee on the bench, your back flat and your head looking down.

● Grip the weight with your palm facing in, ensuring you keep a slight bend in your elbow.

● Raise the weight straight out to the side and lower in a smooth, controlled motion.

⑥ Bench leg raise

Target: **abdominals, hip flexors**

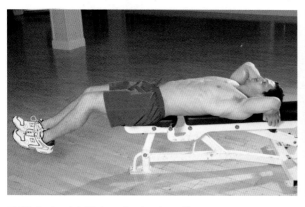
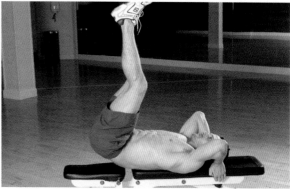

● Grip the bench behind your head, rest your hips on the edge of it and hang your feet over the end.

● Keep your feet together and raise your legs up until they are almost vertical, then use your abs to raise your hips off the bench.

● Reverse the movement to the start in a slow and controlled manner.

WEEK 5
DOING THE SPLITS

WEEK **1**   WEEK **2**   WEEK **3**

Up to this point you've been working on building stability and improving endurance. Now it's time to start packing on muscle.

You'll be doing body-part splits, through which you'll target different muscle groups with each workout, taking your muscles to full exhaustion for the maximum growth effect. You'll start by working your chest, shoulders and triceps in Workout A; legs and glutes in Workout B; and back and biceps in Workout C. Your core and abs will get trained every session thanks to the stabilising requirements of the exercises. The first exercise in each group is designed to fire up your muscles, ready for the heavier weights to come, so keep the resistance manageable for these exercises.

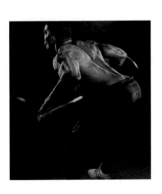

TRAINING PLAN

MON | **WORKOUT A**
(see p82)

TUE | **CARDIO SESSION**
20-minute running intervals
4 minutes warm-up – level 3
30 seconds fast – level 9
1 minute slow – level 4 } x8
4 minutes warm down – level 3

WED | **WORKOUT B**
(see p86)

THU | **REST DAY**

FRI | **WORKOUT C**
(see p90)

SAT | **CARDIO SESSION**
Recovery
Run, swim or cycle at level 5 for 30 minutes, maintaining a steady pace

SUN | **REST DAY**

MEAL PLAN

Breakfast	Snack
4 scrambled egg whites on 2 slices wholemeal toast. 1 grapefruit.	Mixed nuts, raisins and dried cranberries.
Porridge made with 45g oats, 300ml skimmed milk, 1tsp honey and 25g whey protein.	2tbsp peanut butter. 1 apple. Glass of skimmed milk.
2 scrambled eggs on 2 slices of wholemeal toast. 1 grapefruit. Glass of apple juice.	30g brazil nuts. Glass of skimmed milk.
4 scrambled egg whites on 2 slices wholemeal toast. 1 grapefruit.	Mixed nuts, raisins and dried cranberries.
2 scrambled eggs on 2 slices wholemeal toast. Glass of orange juice.	1 mashed banana on 1 piece of wholemeal toast. 1 protein bar.
2 scrambled eggs on 2 slices wholemeal toast. 1 grapefruit. Glass of orange juice.	30g brazil nuts. Glass of skimmed milk.
2 scrambled eggs and baked beans on 2 slices wholemeal toast. Glass of orange juice.	120g low-fat yoghurt with blueberries, honey and oats. 1 protein bar.

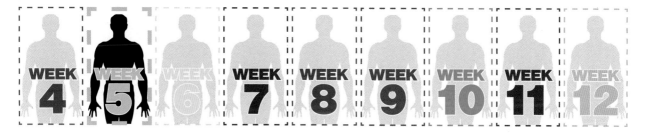

Lunch	Snack	Dinner	Snack	Total
Turkey and cheese bagel. 1 orange.	Smoothie: blend 25g whey protein, 80g strawberries, 80g blueberries and 50g blackberries with 200-300ml water.	20g salmon, with stir-fried broccoli, green beans, red peppers and spinach with sesame oil. 70g brown rice.	Smoothie: blend 25g whey protein, 50g blueberries, 50g blackberries and ½ banana with 300ml skimmed milk.	**2,857 calories** 201g protein 345g carbs 66g fat
Medium-sized jacket potato with tuna, baked beans and grated cheese.	Smoothie: blend 25g whey protein, 80g raspberries, 80g blueberries and 50g blackberries with 200-300ml water.	Steak and lentil casserole (with 300g steak mince, 150g red lentils, garlic, 1 chopped onion, vegetable stock, 2 carrots, 100g mushrooms, 60g aubergine).	120g low-fat yoghurt with strawberries.	**2,945 calories** 210g protein 367g carbs 69g fat
Medium-sized jacket potato with baked beans, tuna and grated cheese.	Smoothie: blend 25g whey protein, 100g strawberries and ½ banana with 300ml skimmed milk and 1tsp flaxseed oil.	150g roast chicken with 100g new potatoes, and mixed vegetables.	100g cottage cheese. 1 apple.	**2,987 calories** 211g protein 361g carbs 73g fat
Turkey and cheese salad sandwich on wholemeal bread. 1 pear.	Smoothie: blend 25g whey protein, 80g raspberries, 80g blueberries and 50g blackberries with water.	200g chicken and vegetable stir fry with red and green peppers, sesame oil and seeds. 70g brown rice.	Smoothie: blend 25g whey protein, 50g blueberries, 50g blackberries and ½ banana with 300ml skimmed milk.	**2,847 calories** 207g protein 345g carbs 65g fat
Turkey salad sandwich on wholemeal bread. 1 apple.	Mixed nuts, raisins and dried cranberries with cottage cheese.	90g wholemeal pasta and 200g grilled chicken with jar of tomato sauce and chopped onion.	Smoothie: blend 25g protein, 50g blueberries, 50g blackberries and ½ banana with 300ml skimmed milk.	**2,835 calories** 211g protein 362g carbs 62g fat
Medium-sized jacket potato with baked beans and cottage cheese.	Smoothie: blend 25g whey protein, 80g raspberries, 80g blueberries and 50g blackberries with water.	150g roast pork with 100g new potatoes and mixed vegetables.	Smoothie: blend, 25g whey protein, 100g strawberries and ½ banana with 1tsp flaxseed oil and 300ml skimmed milk.	**2,995 calories** 211g protein 364g carbs 71g fat
Chicken, bacon and avocado baguette. 1 kiwi.	Smoothie: blend 25g whey protein, ½ banana with 300ml skimmed milk and 1tsp flaxseed oil.	120g tuna steak with stir-fried broccoli, green beans and spinach with sesame oil and seeds. 70g brown rice.	100g cottage cheese and pineapple.	**2,910 calories** 197g protein 364g carbs 67g fat

WORKOUT A

This workout targets your chest, shoulders and triceps. The first exercise warms up your muscles, followed by heavy compound moves to add mass, and the workout ends with isolation moves to take your target muscles to exhaustion.

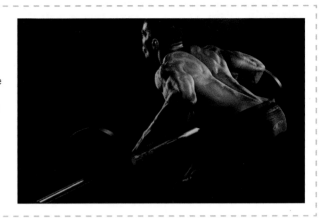

Warm-up Ten minutes of gentle cardio followed by dynamic stretches (see p13)

Exercise		Sets	Reps	Tempo	Rest	Weight
1	Passing medicine ball press-up	2	10	211	45 secs	n/a
2	Incline bench press	4	8-10	311	60 secs	
3	Feet up bench dip	3	10-12	211	45 secs	n/a
4	Seated dumb-bell shoulder press	4	8-10	311	60 secs	
5	Lying triceps extension	3	10-12	311	45 secs	
6	Cable crossover	3	10-12	311	45 secs	

Warm down and stretch Ten minutes of gentle cardio plus static stretches (20 seconds each). Focus on chest, triceps, shoulders (see p14)

Notes

① **Passing medicine ball press-up**

Target: pecs, triceps

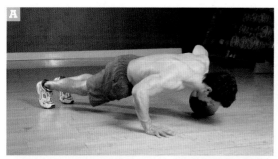

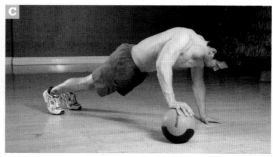

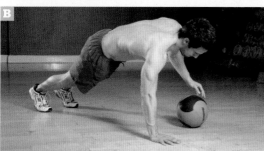

- Start with your feet shoulder width apart, one hand on a medicine ball and the other on the floor.
- Keep your body straight from head to heels and don't let your hips sag.
- Perform a press-up, push up and pass the medicine ball to the other hand and repeat the movement.
- Pass the ball back and forth with each press-up.

② **Incline bench press**

Target: upper pecs, front deltoids, triceps

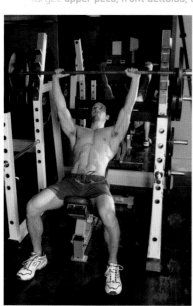

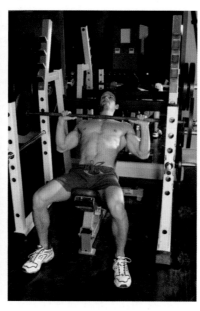

- Set the bench at 30-45°, keep your feet flat on the floor and grip the bar slightly wider than shoulder width apart.
- Brace your core, remove the bar from the rack and hold it directly above your chest.
- Lower the bar slowly to your chest and press up powerfully, keep your elbows to the sides and don't arch your back.

3 Feet up bench dip

Target: triceps

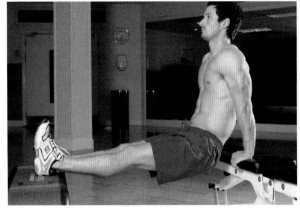 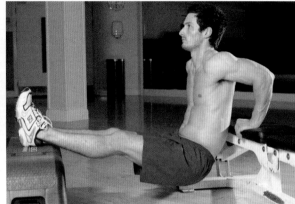

● Grip the edge of the bench with your palms facing back.

● Place your feet on a bench of the same height with your legs straight and your feet together.

● Keeping your back upright, lower your body straight down, keeping your elbows pointing back, then press back up powerfully.

4 Seated dumb-bell shoulder press

Target: deltoids

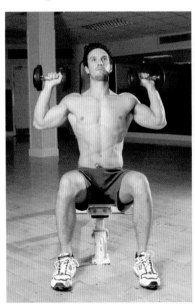 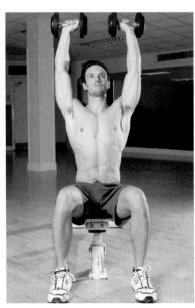

● Sit on a bench with your lower back and shoulders pressed against the pad.

● Keeping your feet flat on the floor, hold the dumb-bells at shoulder height with your elbows out to the sides.

● Press the weights directly overhead but don't let them touch at the top, lower slowly.

● Keep your core braced throughout and don't arch your back.

⑤ Lying triceps extension

Target: **triceps**

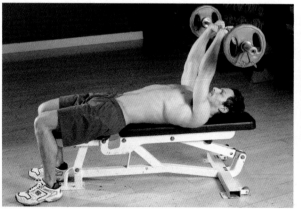 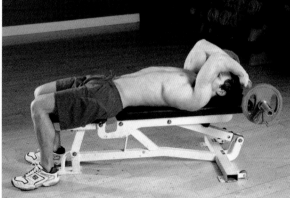

● Lie on a bench with your core braced, knees bent at 90° and feet flat on the ground.

● Hold the EZ-bar over your head, not your chest, with an overhand grip, wrists turned in slightly.

● Without arching your back

lower the bar slowly behind your head while keeping your upper arms angled slightly back.

● Reverse the motion to press the bar back up, squeezing your triceps at the top of the move.

⑥ Cable crossover

Target: **pecs**

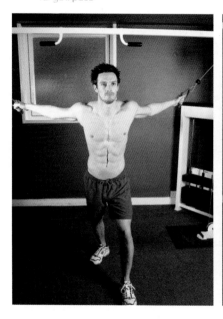 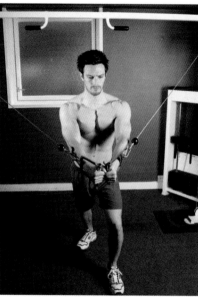

● Stand in a split stance, between dual cables set above shoulder height.

● Keep your back upright and your core braced, maintaining the same torso position throughout.

● Keep a slight bend in your elbows and bring your hands together in front of your chest. Squeeze your pecs then slowly reverse the move.

WORKOUT B

This workout targets your legs and glutes. The first exercise warms up your muscles, then you'll move on to the heavy compound moves to add mass, and finish off with moves to target the smaller muscles that often get ignored.

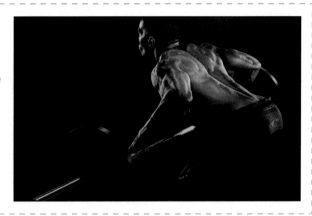

Warm-up Ten minutes of gentle cardio followed by dynamic stretches (see p13)

Exercise		Sets	Reps	Tempo	Rest	Weight
1	Gym ball Bulgarian split squat	2	**8** each leg	311	30 secs	
2	Squat	4	8-10	311	60 secs	
3	Lateral lunge	3	**6** each side	311	45 secs	
4	Romanian deadlift	4	8-10	311	60 secs	
5	Gym ball hip raise	3	10-12	311	45 secs	n/a
6	Standing calf raise	3	10-12	311	45 secs	

Warm down and stretch Ten minutes of gentle cardio plus static stretches (20 seconds each). Focus on quads, glutes, hams, hip flexors, adductors, calves (see p14)

Notes

① Gym ball Bulgarian split squat

Target: quads, glutes

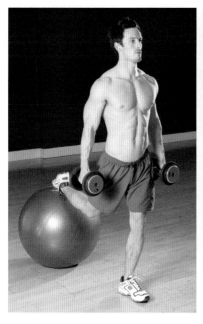
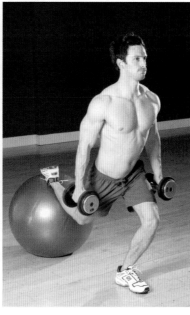

● Rest the instep of your back foot on the ball and plant the other foot flat on the floor, facing forwards, half a metre or so in front of the ball.

● Keep your torso upright, your core braced and your hips facing forwards.

● Lower until your front thigh is almost parallel to the floor.

● Keep your front knee in line with your foot but make sure it doesn't travel beyond your toes.

② Squat

Target quads, glutes, hamstrings

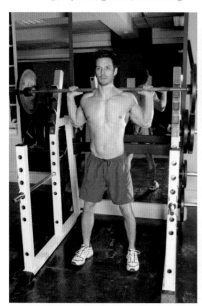
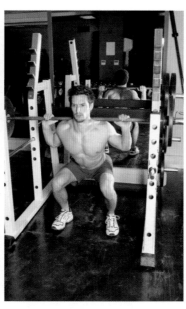

● Stand with your feet shoulder width apart, your toes turned out slightly and your core braced.

● Rest the bar on the back of your shoulders, not your neck, gripping it close to your shoulders.

● Maintain a natural arch in your back and look forward throughout the movement.

● Lower until your thighs are parallel to the floor, keeping your knees in line with your feet, then push back up through your heels.

③ Lateral lunge

Target: adductors, quads

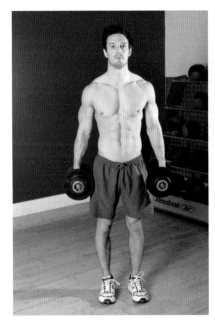 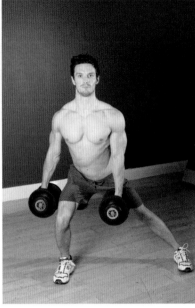

- Stand with your feet close together, your torso upright and your head facing forward.
- Take a big step to one side and lower onto your leading leg, keeping the other leg straight.
- Keep your feet pointing forward and your leading knee in line with your foot.
- Push back from your leading leg to return to the start.

④ Romanian deadlift

Target: hamstrings

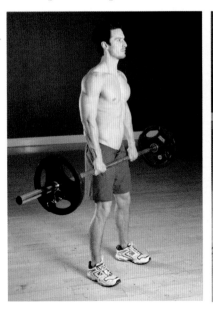 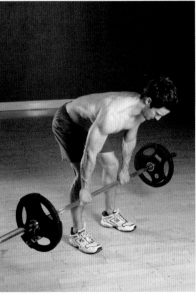

- Stand with your feet shoulder width apart and your head up.
- Keep looking forward, with your shoulders back and core braced.
- Grip the bar just outside your hips and initiate the move by leaning forward from the hips rather than the waist.
- Allow a slight bend in your knees, keep your back straight and push your hips back as the bar travels down your shins.
- Lower the bar until you feel a good stretch in your hamstrings then reverse the movement to the start.

⑤ **Gym ball hip raise**

Target: hip flexors, core

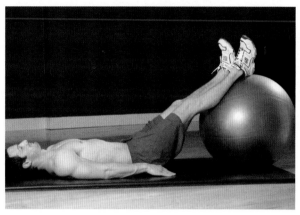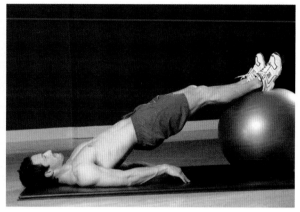

● Start with your body flat on the floor, your heels resting on top of the ball and your arms by your sides.

● Brace your core and raise your hips until your body is straight from shoulders to heels.

● Hold for 10-12 seconds.

⑥ **Standing calf raise**

Target: calves

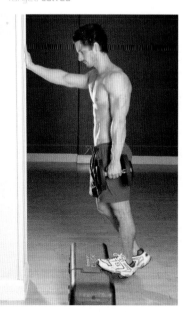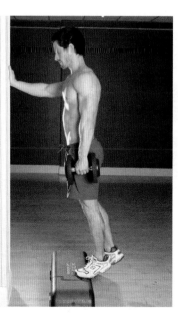

● Place the ball of your foot on the edge of a step with your heel down, allow the non-working foot to hang free.

● Keep your body upright and with your free hand hold a wall for balance.

● Push up until your heel is as high as it can go, hold and squeeze the calf for a moment before lowering slowly.

WORKOUT C

In this workout you'll focus on your back and biceps, which are often called on to work together when pulling objects towards you. The first exercise will get the muscles fired up before the heavy compound moves that follow.

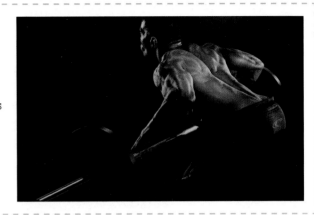

Warm-up Ten minutes of gentle cardio followed by dynamic stretches (see p13)

Exercise		Sets	Reps	Tempo	Rest	Weight
1 Split squat to one-arm row		2	10-12 each side	311	30 secs	
2 Cable row		4	8-10	311	60 secs	
3 Pull-up		4	6-10	311	60 secs	n/a
4 Dumb-bell curl		3	10-12	311	45 secs	
5 Dumb-bell shrug		4	8-10	311	60 secs	
6 Reverse curl		3	10-12	311	45 secs	

Warm down and stretch Ten minutes of gentle cardio plus static stretches (20 seconds each). Focus on lats, traps, lower back, biceps (see p14)

Notes

❶ Split squat to one-arm row

Target: legs, back, arms, shoulders, core

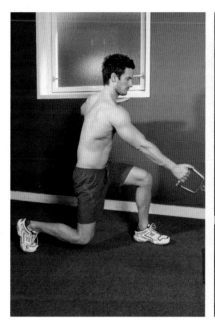 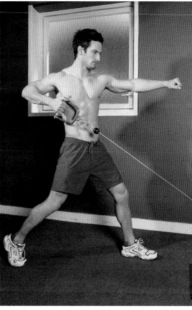

● Start in a lunge position with your left leg forward and your right hand gripping a low cable handle.

● Turn your body towards the cable, keep your head upright and your core braced.

● Stand up, draw the cable back to your side and retract your shoulder blade while turning your body away from the cable.

❷ Cable row

Target: mid traps, lats, rhomboids

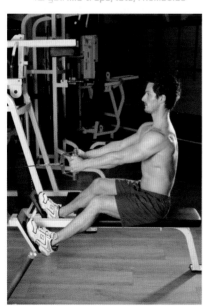 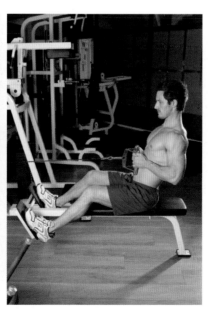

● Sit with a slight bend in your knees, your back straight, shoulder blades retracted and head looking forward.

● Take a neutral grip on the handle and ensure that there is tension in the cable.

● Keeping upper-body movement to a minimum, pull the handle into your sternum and squeeze your shoulder blades together.

● Return in a slow and controlled manner.

③ Pull-up

Target: lats, traps, rhomboids

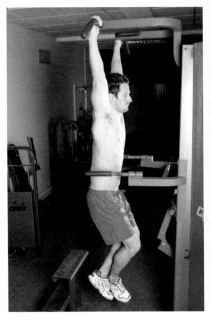 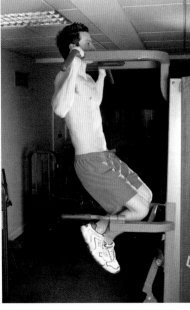

● Grip the bar with an overhand grip, just wider than shoulder width apart.

● Extend your arms fully, letting your body hang straight down without swinging.

● Pull up until your chin is over the bar, squeezing your lats as you rise.

● Lower slowly without swinging.

④ Dumb-bell curl

Target: biceps

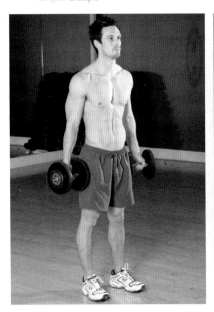 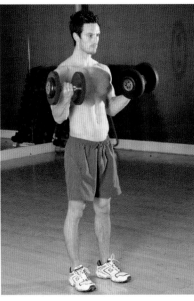

● Stand tall with your shoulders back and your core muscles braced for support.

● Keep your elbows tucked into your sides and grip the dumb-bells with your palms facing forwards.

● Curl the weights up without rocking back and forth for momentum, then lower slowly.

⑤ Dumb-bell shrug

Target upper traps

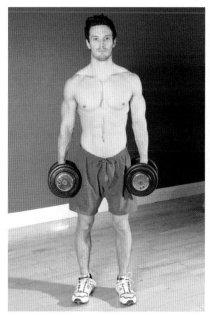 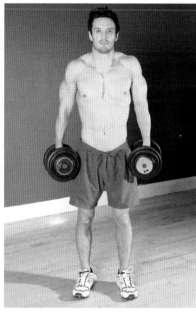

● Stand upright with your shoulders back, gripping the dumb-bells with your palms facing in.

● Without bending your elbows, raise your shoulders straight up and hold for 1-2 seconds.

⑥ Reverse curl

Target: biceps

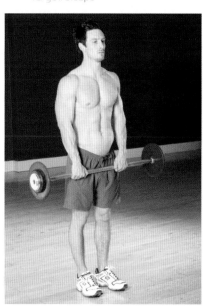 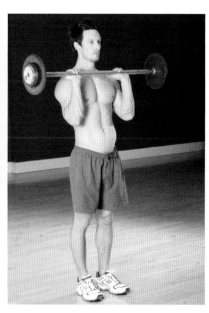

● Stand tall with your shoulders back and your core muscles braced for support.

● Grip the bar with an overhand grip, in front of your thighs.

● Keeping your elbows in, curl the bar up without rocking back and forth for momentum, then lower slowly.

WEEK 6
HITTING THE POST

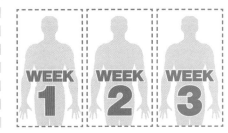

WEEK 1 WEEK 2 WEEK 3

In week six you'll use the power of 'post-exhaustion' to stimulate muscle growth. This classic weight-training technique requires you to target a particular muscle group with a big, compound move to stress the maximum number of muscle fibres and flood the body with growth hormones. Then you'll zero in on your target muscle with a single-joint or isolation move to take those muscle fibres to exhaustion.

In Workout A you'll target your chest, back and quads; Workout B is shoulders, biceps and hamstrings; while Workout C hits your triceps, traps and glutes.

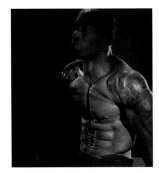

TRAINING PLAN

MON

WORKOUT A
(see p96)

TUE

CARDIO SESSION
Running hill intervals
Run up a steep hill or long set of steps for 1 minute. Jog down again slowly. Repeat 6 times. Afterwards run at level 3 for 5 minutes to warm down

WED

WORKOUT B
(see p100)

THU

REST DAY

FRI

WORKOUT C
(see p104)

SAT

CARDIO SESSION
Recovery
Run, swim or cycle at level 5 for 30 minutes, maintaining a steady pace

SUN

REST DAY

MEAL PLAN

Breakfast	Snack
2 slices French toast made with 1 egg, 110ml milk, ½tsp cinnamon and ½tsp nutmeg.	120g low-fat yoghurt with blueberries, honey and oats. 1 protein bar.
Porridge, made with 45g oats, 300ml skimmed milk, 1tsp honey and 25g whey protein.	1 mashed banana with 2tbsp peanut butter on 2 slices wholemeal toast.
2 slices French toast made with 1 egg, 110ml milk, ½tsp cinnamon and ½tsp nutmeg.	120g low-fat yoghurt with blueberries, honey and oats. 1 protein bar.
Porridge made with 45g oats, 300ml skimmed milk, 1tsp of honey and 25g whey protein.	1 mashed banana with 2tbsp peanut butter on 2 slices wholemeal toast.
Porridge made with 45g oats, 300ml skimmed milk, 1tsp of honey and 25g whey protein.	1 mashed banana on 1 slice wholemeal toast.
Porridge made with 45g oats with 300ml skimmed milk, 1tsp of honey and 25g whey protein.	90g mackerel on 2 slices wholemeal toast. Glass of skimmed milk.
Smoothie: blend 25g whey protein, 1 mango, 80g blueberries, 2tbsp natural yoghurt and 1tbsp oats with 100ml apple juice and 100ml water.	90g sardines with lemon juice on 2 slices wholemeal toast.

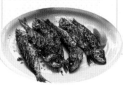

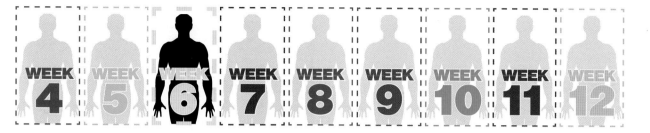
Lunch	Snack	Dinner	Snack	Total
Chicken, bacon and avocado baguette. 1 pear.	Smoothie: blend 25g whey protein, 100g strawberries and ½ banana with 300ml skimmed milk and 1tsp flaxseed oil.	120g tuna steak, with stir-fried broccoli, green beans and spinach with sesame oil and seeds. 70g brown rice.	100g cottage cheese and pineapple.	**2,831 calories** 200g protein 362g carbs 67g fat
Turkey, cheese and mustard bagel. 1 apple.	1 tin of tuna with beetroot. 125g low-fat yoghurt.	120g fillet steak with mashed potato and spinach. Fruit sorbet.	Smoothie: blend 25g whey protein, 80g raspberries, 80g blueberries and 50g blackberries with 200-300ml water.	**2,950 calories** 210g protein 359g carbs 68g fat
Turkey and cranberry wholemeal sandwich. Punnet of berries.	Smoothie: blend 25g whey protein, 100g strawberries and ½ banana with 300ml skimmed milk and 1tsp flaxseed oil.	150g lean minced beef chilli with red kidney beans. 70g brown rice.	100g cottage cheese and pineapple.	**2,837 calories** 208g protein 372g carbs 67g fat
Turkey, cheese and mustard bagel. 1 low-fat yoghurt.	1 tin of tuna with beetroot. 1 pear.	120g fillet steak with mashed potato and spinach. Slice of cheesecake.	Smoothie: blend 25g whey protein, 80g raspberries, 80g blueberries and 50g blackberries with 200-300ml water.	**2,985 calories** 209g protein 369g carbs 74g fat
Turkey salad sandwich on wholemeal bread. 1 orange.	Mixed nuts, raisins and dried cranberries with cottage cheese.	150g lean minced beef spaghetti bolognese with chopped onions, peppers and mushrooms. 70g wholemeal spaghetti.	Smoothie: blend 25g protein, 50g blueberries, 50g blackberries ½ banana with 300ml skimmed milk.	**2,895 calories** 204g protein 363g carbs 65g fat
Large jacket potato with tuna, baked beans and grated cheese.	Smoothie: blend 25g whey protein, 80g raspberries, 80g blueberries and 50g blackberries with 200-300ml water.	Omelette with ham, feta cheese, olives, tomato and onion.	120g low-fat yoghurt with strawberries.	**2,982 calories** 184g protein 327g carbs 67g fat
Large jacket potato with baked beans and cottage cheese.	140g grilled chicken with beetroot.	200g chicken and vegetable stir-fry with red and green peppers, cashew nuts, sesame oil and seeds. 70g brown rice.	Smoothie: blend 25g whey protein, 80g raspberries, 80g blueberries and 50g blackberries with 200-300ml water.	**2,903 calories** 198g protein 365g carbs 69g fat

WORKOUT A

This workout is for your chest, back and quads using post-exhaustion techniques. For each muscle group you'll do a heavy compound exercise that requires a lot of muscle fibres and floods your body with growth hormones, then you'll take the muscle to exhaustion with a move that targets it specifically.

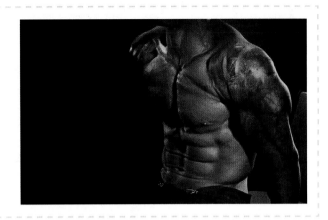

Warm-up Ten minutes of gentle cardio followed by dynamic stretches (see p13)

Exercise		Sets	Reps	Tempo	Rest	Weight
① Bench press		4	8-10	311	60 secs	
② Dumb-bell flye		3	10-12	311	45 secs	
③ Bent-over row		4	8-10	311	60 secs	
④ Cable reverse flye		3	10-12	311	45 secs	
⑤ Cross-grip front squat		4	8-10	311	60 secs	
⑥ One-leg Smith squat		3	6 each side	311	45 secs	

Warm down and stretch Ten minutes of gentle cardio plus static stretches (20 seconds each). Focus on chest, triceps, traps, biceps, quads, glutes, lower back (see p14)

Notes

① Bench press

Target pecs, triceps

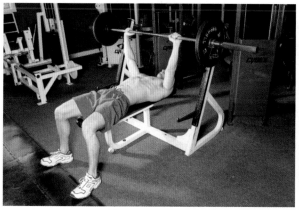 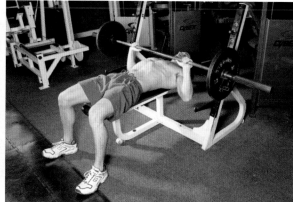

- Lie on the bench with your knees bent at 90°, your feet flat on the floor and your core braced.

- Grip the bar wider than shoulder width, retract your shoulder blades and lift the bar off the rack, holding it directly over your chest.

- Maintain a natural arch in your back. There should just be enough room to slip a few fingers between your lower back and the bench.

- Lower the bar to your chest slowly and press up powerfully.

② Dumb-bell flye

Target pecs

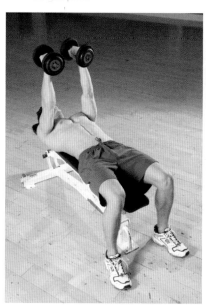 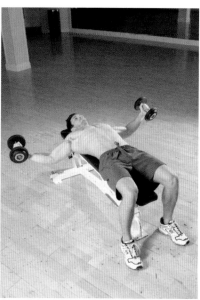

- Lie on a bench with your feet flat on the floor.

- Hold the dumb-bells directly over your chest with your palms facing each other, keeping a slight bend in your elbows.

- Without arching your back, lower the dumb-bells in an arc out to the sides as far as is comfortable.

- Use your pectoral muscles to reverse the movement back to the start.

③ Bent-over row
Target: traps, lats, rhomboids

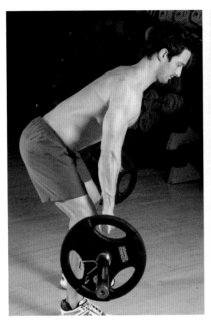
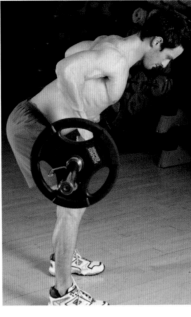

⦿ Start with your core braced, your back straight and your shoulder blades retracted.

⦿ With your knees slightly bent, lean forward from the hips, rather than the waist, keep your back straight.

⦿ Grip the bar just wider than shoulder width apart, letting it hang straight down around knee level.

⦿ Pull the bar up into your sternum, squeezing your shoulder blades together at the top of the move, then lower the bar slowly to the start.

④ Cable reverse flye
Target: rear deltoids, back

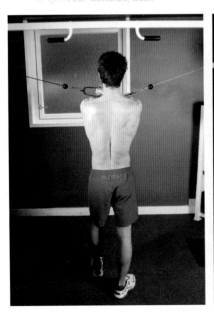
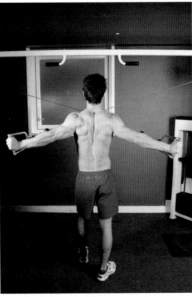

⦿ Stand in a split stance between twin high cables, holding the handles with your arms straight and crossed over.

⦿ Brace your core, keep your arms straight and your hands high.

⦿ Without leaning back, pull the cables straight out and squeeze your shoulder blades together before slowly reversing the move.

⑤ Cross-grip front squat

Target: quads, glutes

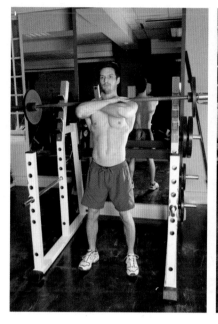
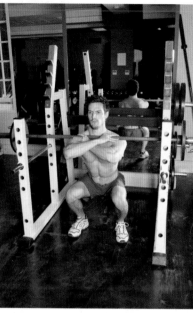

● Stand with your feet shoulder width apart, your toes turned out slightly and your core braced.

● Rest the bar on the front of your shoulders, cross your arms and grip it with your fingertips.

● Keeping your elbows high, maintain a natural arch in your back and look forward throughout the movement.

● Lower until your thighs are parallel to the floor, keeping your knees in line with your feet, then push back up through your heels.

⑥ One-leg Smith squat

Target: quads, glutes

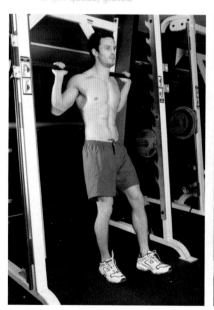
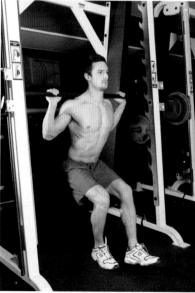

● Place one foot slightly in front of your body to put more emphasis on your quads, keep the other foot off the floor.

● Rest the bar on the back of your shoulders, not your neck, look forward and brace your core.

● Unlock the bar from the rack and lower as far as feels comfortable, then push back up through your heel.

WORKOUT B

This session will work your shoulders, hamstrings and biceps. Once again you'll start with mass-building compound exercises and follow them with isolation moves to stimulate the maximum muscle growth.

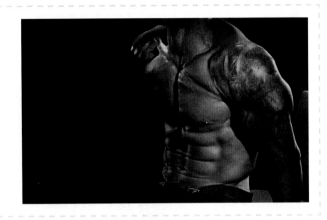

Warm-up Ten minutes of gentle cardio followed by dynamic stretches (see p13)

Exercise		Sets	Reps	Tempo	Rest	Weight
① Romanian deadlift		4	8-10	311	60 secs	
② One-leg gym ball leg curl		3	8 each leg	311	45 secs	n/a
③ Shoulder press		4	8-10	311	60 secs	
④ Lateral raise		3	10-12	311	45 secs	
⑤ Chin-up		4	5-10	311	60 secs	n/a
⑥ EZ-bar biceps curl		3	10-12	311	45 secs	

Warm down and stretch Ten minutes of gentle cardio plus static stretches (20 seconds each). Focus on hams, glutes, shoulders, biceps, lats (see p14)

Notes

① Romanian deadlift

Target: hamstrings

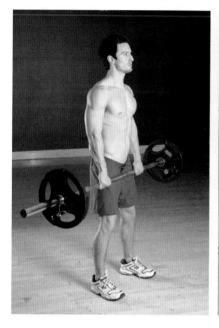 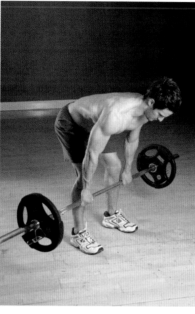

● Stand with your feet shoulder width apart and your head up.

● Keep looking forward, with your shoulders back and core braced.

● Grip the bar just outside your hips and initiate the move by leaning forward from the hips rather than the waist.

● Allow a slight bend in your knees, keep your back straight and push your hips back as the bar travels down your shins.

● Lower the bar until you feel a good stretch in your hamstrings then reverse the movement to the start.

② One-leg gym ball leg curl

Target: hamstrings

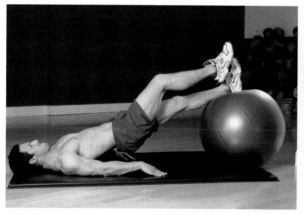 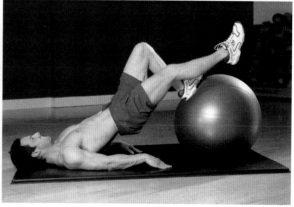

● Rest your head and shoulders on the mat, place one heel on the ball and hold the other slightly raised.

● Keep your body straight from shoulders to heels and your arms by your sides.

● Curl the ball in towards your backside using your heel, keep your hips raised, pause at the top of the movement and return under control.

③ Shoulder press
Target: deltoids

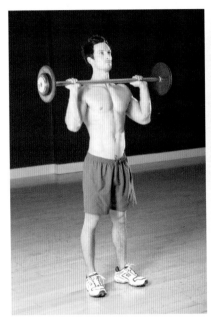
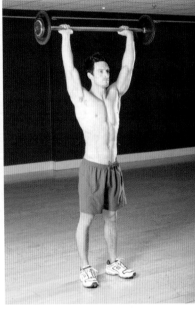

● Stand with your feet shoulder width apart, your body upright, core braced and head looking straight ahead.

● Grip the bar just wider than shoulder width apart and hold it on your upper chest.

● Press the bar directly overhead without tilting your hips forward, slowly lower it to the start.

④ Lateral raise
Target: middle deltoid

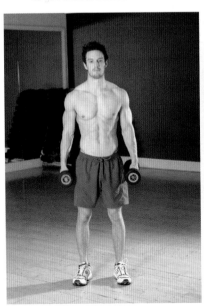
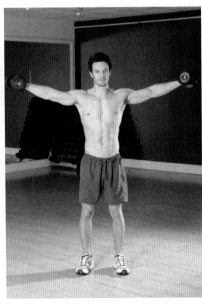

● Stand with your feet shoulder width apart, body upright and core braced.

● Use light dumb-bells, with your palms facing in.

● Keeping your arms straight, lift the weights out to the sides but don't swing your body for momentum.

● Stop lifting at shoulder height and hold for a moment before lowering slowly.

⑤ Chin-up

Target: biceps, lats

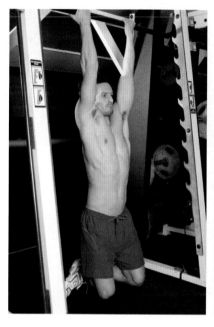
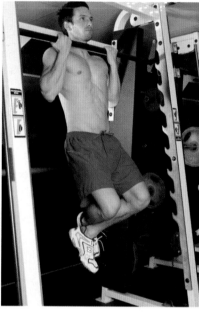

● Grasp the bar with an underhand grip, hands shoulder width apart.

● Lower until your arms are fully extended, cross your legs behind you and try not to swing.

● Pull up until your chin is over the bar and squeeze your biceps hard at the top of the move.

● Lower slowly to the start without swinging.

⑥ EZ-bar biceps curl

Target: biceps

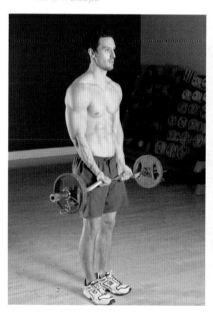
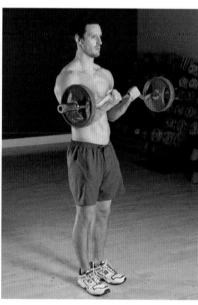

● Stand tall with your shoulders back and your core muscles braced for support.

● Keep your elbows tucked into your sides and grip the EZ-bar with your hands turned inwards slightly.

● Lift the bar without rocking back and forth for momentum, stop before your forearms are vertical and lower slowly.

WORKOUT C

Target your triceps, traps and glutes. These large muscle groups will stimulate a surge in growth hormones that will have a muscle-building effect on all parts of your body.

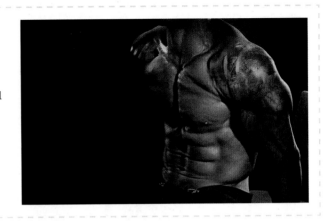

Warm-up Ten minutes of gentle cardio followed by dynamic stretches (see p13)

Exercise		Sets	Reps	Tempo	Rest	Weight
1 Deadlift		4	8-10	311	60 secs	
2 One-leg gym ball hip raise		3	8 each leg	311	45 secs	n/a
3 Upright row		4	8-10	311	60 secs	
4 Prone shoulder press		3	10-12	311	45 secs	
5 Dip		4	8-10	311	60 secs	n/a
6 Rope press down		3	10-12	311	45 secs	

Warm down and stretch Ten minutes of gentle cardio plus static stretches (20 seconds each). Focus on hams, glutes, traps, triceps, lower back, hip flexors (see p14)

Notes

① Deadlift

Target: quads, glutes, hamstrings, back, core

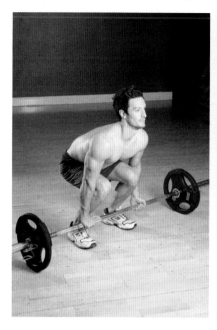
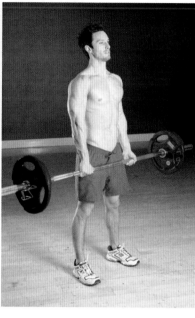

● Start with your feet shoulder width apart, grasp the bar outside your knees with an overhand or alternate grip.

● Position the bar close to your shins with your shoulders directly over it and keep looking forward.

● Ensure you keep your back flat, your shoulders retracted and your core braced.

● Start the lift by pushing with your glutes and pushing down through the heels.

● Keeping your shoulders back, the bar should rise up your shins. As it passes your knees, push your hips forward.

② One-leg gym ball hip raise

Target: hip flexors, core

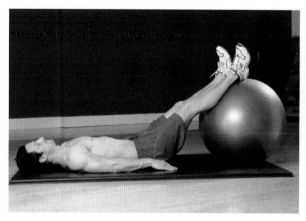
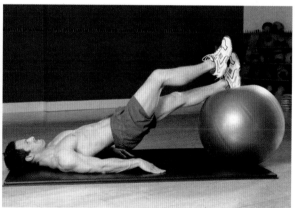

● Start with your body flat on the floor and your arms by your sides.

● Rest your heels on top of the ball, then raise one foot slightly.

● Brace your core then raise your hips until your body is straight from shoulders to heels.

● Control any wobble from the ball and lower slowly to the start.

③ Upright row

Target: upper traps, deltoids

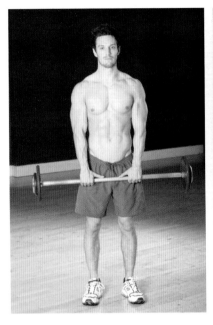 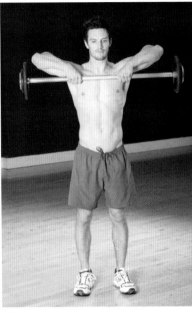

- Stand upright with your shoulders back, gripping the bar in front of your thighs.
- Brace your core and draw the weight up, raising your elbows high to the sides.
- Pause for a moment at the top of the movement before slowly lowering.

④ Prone shoulder press

Target: traps, deltoids

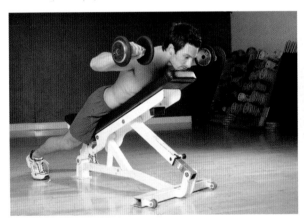 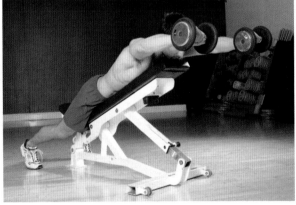

- Lie face down on a bench set at 30-45°.
- Position your upper arms straight out from your body with your elbows bent at 90° and your forearms in line with your body, similar to a shoulder press but prone.
- Press the weights straight out ahead of you. Return in a controlled manner.

⑤ Dip
Target: triceps, chest

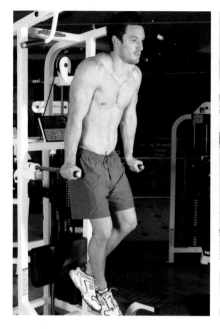
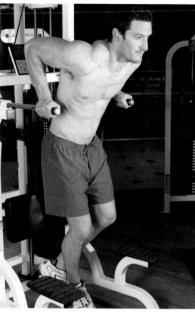

● Grip parallel bars just wider than hip width. Keep your body straight.

● Keeping your elbows straight back, lower yourself slowly as far as is comfortable.

● Push back up powerfully, don't swing your legs for momentum.

⑥ Rope press down
Target: triceps

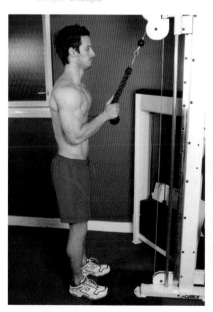
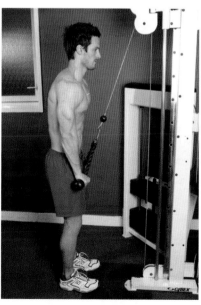

● Stand in front of a cable set at head height. If it helps your balance then place one foot in front of the other.

● Grasp a rope attachment using a hammer grip. Keep your back straight and your elbows tucked in throughout the movement.

● Without leaning forward press the weight down, turn your wrists out at the bottom of the move and squeeze your triceps.

WEEK 7
DOING THE DROP

You're now ready to give your muscles a bit of a shock. Drop sets are when you do one regular set of an exercise to failure then immediately strip off some weight and do as many reps as you can, before reducing the weight again and continuing until your muscles are completely exhausted. Your body will respond to this punishment by getting bigger and stronger as you recover afterwards.

Because they're such a shock to the system, drop sets aren't a good idea for every workout, and you'll only do one drop-set exercise per workout this week.

This week's splits are back, biceps and core for Workout A; chest, triceps and core for Workout B; legs, shoulders and core for Workout C.

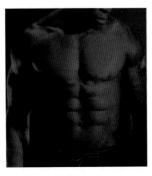

TRAINING PLAN

MON	**WORKOUT A** (see p110)
TUE	**CARDIO SESSION** 20-minute running intervals 4 minutes warm-up – level 3 2 minutes fast – level 7 } x3 2 minutes slow – level 4 4 minutes warm down – level 3
WED	**WORKOUT B** (see p114)
THU	**REST DAY**
FRI	**WORKOUT C** (see p118)
SAT	**CARDIO SESSION** Recovery Run, swim or cycle at level 5 for 40 minutes, maintaining a steady pace
SUN	**REST DAY**

MEAL PLAN

Breakfast	Snack
75g oats cooked in water. 1 banana and a handful of raisins.	50g beef jerky. 1 apple.
Cook 100g oats in water. When cooked, add 100g blackberries and stir for 2 minutes. Top with 1tbsp pumpkin seeds and 1tbsp honey.	150g natural yoghurt. 1 energy bar.
60g muesli with 200ml semi-skimmed milk and 25g mixed dried fruit and nuts. 200ml orange juice.	Smoothie: blend 50ml apple juice 1 peach, ½ punnet of strawberries, 1tsp honey, 75g natural yoghurt. Oatmeal flapjack.
2 slices wholemeal toast with 1 large mashed banana, 5tsp peanut butter and a sprinkling of grated coconut.	50g beef jerky. 2 hard-boiled eggs. 1 pear.
Chop 1 apple, 1 pear, 1 banana and 1 peach. Serve with juice of ½ lime and 2tsp chopped almonds, 2tsp pecan nuts, 2tsp pumpkin seeds and 2tsp raisins.	1 toasted wholemeal pitta, 2tsp chickpeas, 100g low-fat cottage cheese and salad.
2 rashers of bacon, 2 sausages, 2 slices of wholemeal toast, black pudding, baked beans and 2 grilled tomatoes.	Smoothie: blend 50ml apple juice, 1 banana, ½ punnet of raspberries, 1tsp flaked almonds, 100ml natural yoghurt
2 slices of thin-cut raw, fresh salmon, 3 scrambled eggs and 1 slice of sourdough toast.	2 rye crackers with generous serving of chicken-liver pâté.

| WEEK | WEEK | WEEK | WEEK | WEEK | WEEK | WEEK | WEEK | WEEK |
| 4 | 5 | 6 | 7 | 8 | 9 | 10 | 11 | 12 |

Lunch	Snack	Dinner	Snack	Total
Greek salad (tomatoes, cucumber, ½ yellow pepper, black olives, 60g feta cheese, 1 tin of tuna, cider vinegar). 1 wholemeal pitta.	200g low-fat fruit yoghurt.	Grilled cod fillet with 1 courgette, 100g mangetout, 100g cauliflower, 100g wholemeal pasta.	50g almonds and 100g grapes.	**2,970 calories,** 176g protein, 288g carbs, 139g fat
2 chicken sandwiches: 1 chicken breast, 2 handfuls of salad leaves, handful of fresh coriander, ½ sliced avocado, 2 sliced tomatoes, 1 sliced hard-boiled egg and 5 slices of cucumber on wholemeal bread.	30g sunflower seeds. 1 large apple.	1 sliced skinless chicken breast stir-fried with ginger, 1 sliced courgette, 1 sliced carrot, sugar snap peas and soy sauce. Serve with 75g quinoa.	1 banana. 30g sunflower seeds.	**3,013 calories,** 156g protein, 388g carbs, 99g fat
1 tin of vegetable soup and 1 wholemeal baguette.	1 banana. 50g mixed nuts.	225g sirloin steak, 2 sweet potatoes, mixed vegetables and corn on the cob.	200ml vanilla ice cream.	**2,961 calories,** 141g protein, 409g carbs, 135g fat
300g mixed seafood salad (tuna, prawns, salmon, anchovies) and 150g rice.	35g cheddar cheese, 1 apple, 2 pineapple rings.	Stir-fry 4 cauliflower florets, 4 broccoli florets and 100g green beans with sesame oil, soy sauce and chopped ginger. Serve with 75g quinoa and 1 grilled turkey breast.	200g yoghurt with a handful of mixed berries.	**2,840 calories** 305g protein 171g carbs 104g fat
Baked potato with 1 small tin of salmon, ½ avocado, baby spinach, watercress and balsamic vinegar.	½ carton of fresh soup. ½ banana.	1 grilled tuna steak, 75g basmati rice and stir-fried mangetout, baby corn and carrots.	150g natural yoghurt with ½ banana and 1tsp honey.	**2,941 calories** 164g protein 371g carbs 95g fat
Sardines and salad in 2 wholemeal pitta breads.	50g dried fruit and nuts.	Breaded plaice and 125g oven-roasted chips with mushy peas.	Protein shake with 200ml semi-skimmed milk.	**2,900 calories,** 161g protein, 272g carbs, 156g fat
1 tin of mixed beans with 25g goat's cheese and seasoning. 1 slice of wholemeal bread with butter. 1 banana.	50g mixed nuts. 1 apple. 1 pear.	2 chicken breasts with jerk sauce, 150g rice and peas.	3tsp peanut butter. 1 banana.	**2,800 calories,** 310g protein, 163g carbs, 101g fat

WORKOUT A

For your first workout of week seven, you'll focus on the muscles of your back, biceps and core. Look out for the drop sets on the cable row, where you'll do one set of 10-12 reps and then immediately drop the weight by around 20 per cent and then do as many more reps as you can to failure. Then drop the weight again and repeat the process four or five times until your muscles are fully exhausted.

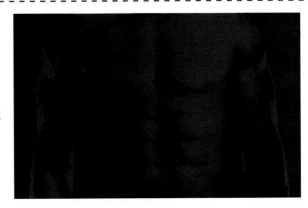

Warm-up Ten minutes of gentle cardio followed by dynamic stretches (see p13)

Exercise		Sets	Reps	Tempo	Rest	Weight
1 Wide grip pull-up		2	5-10	311	60 secs	n/a
2 Snatch grip deadlift		3	8-10	311	60 secs	
3 Cable row		1 drop set	10-12 (+ as many more as possible)	311	60 secs	
4 Rope cable curl		3	10-12	311	60 secs	
5 Jackknife		3	10-12	211	60 secs	n/a
6 Aquaman		2	10-12	202	60 secs	n/a

Warm down and stretch Ten minutes of gentle cardio plus static stretches (20 seconds each). Focus on glutes, abs, traps, lats, biceps, abs, lower back (see p14)

Notes

❶ Wide grip pull-up

Target: lats, traps, rhomboids

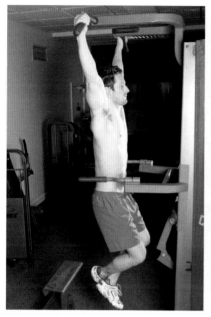 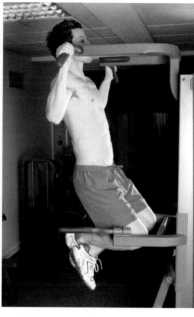

● Grip the bar with a wide, overhand grip.

● Extend your arms fully, letting your body hang straight down without swinging.

● Pull up until your chin is over the bar, squeezing your lats as you do.

● Lower slowly without swinging.

❷ Snatch grip deadlift

Target: back, quads, glutes, hamstrings, core

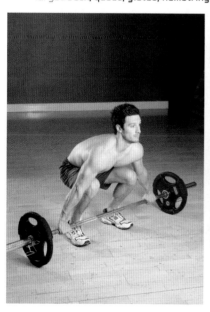 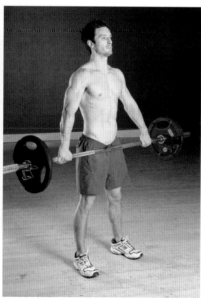

● Start with your feet shoulder width apart and grasp the bar with a wide, overhand grip.

● Position the bar close to your shins with your shoulders directly over it and keep looking forward.

● Ensure you keep your back flat, your shoulders retracted and your core braced.

● Start the lift by pushing with your glutes and pushing down through your heels.

● Keeping your shoulders back, the bar should rise up your shins, as it passes your knees, push your hips forward.

3 Cable row

Target: **mid traps, lats, rhomboids**

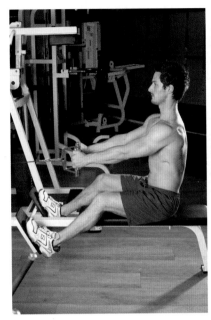
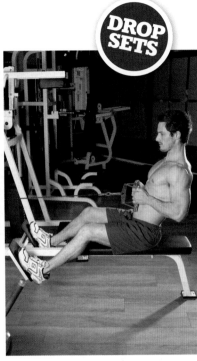

DROP SETS

● Sit with a slight bend in your knees, your back straight, shoulder blades retracted and head looking forward.

● Take a neutral grip on the bar and ensure that there is tension in the cable.

● Keeping upper-body movement to a minimum, pull the bar into your sternum and squeeze your shoulder blades together.

● Return in a slow and controlled manner.

4 Rope cable curl

Target: **biceps**

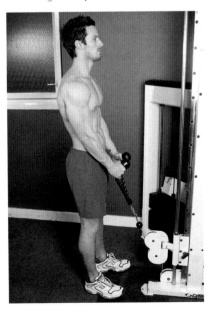
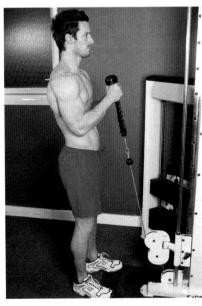

● Stand tall with your shoulders back and your core muscles braced for support.

● Grasp a rope attachment with a hammer grip and keep your elbows tucked into your sides.

● Lift the weight without leaning back, stop before your forearms are vertical and lower slowly.

⑤ Jackknife

Target: **upper and lower abdominals**

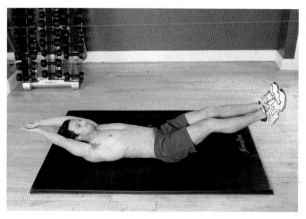
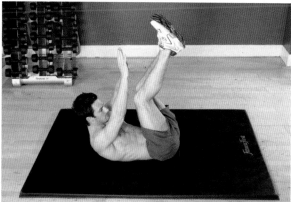

● Start with your arms behind your head, held off the floor, and your feet together, also off the floor.

● Contract your abs to bring your arms and legs up to meet above your stomach, keep your legs as straight as you can.

● Squeeze your abs hard at the top of the move and lower to the start slowly.

⑥ Aquaman

Target: **lower back**

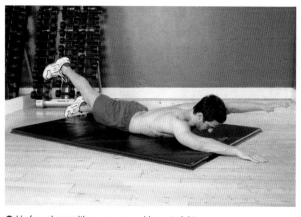
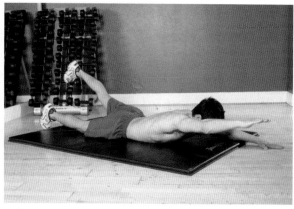

● Lie face down with your arms and legs straight and your head raised slightly off the floor.

● Lift one arm and the opposite leg, keeping both of them straight.

● Lower and repeat the movement with the alternate arm and leg.

WORKOUT B

Target your chest, triceps and core in this workout. Your drop-set session will be with the dumb-bell bench press, so keep a selection of weights near your bench so that you don't have to keep making trips to the weight rack to change the dumb-bells.

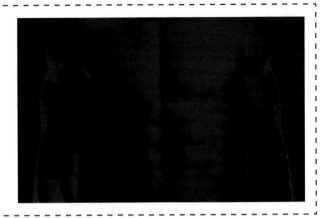

Warm-up Ten minutes of gentle cardio followed by dynamic stretches (see p13)

Exercise		Sets	Reps	Tempo	Rest	Weight
❶ T press-up		2	10-12	31X	60 secs	
❷ Cable pullover		3	10-12	311	60 secs	
❸ Dumb-bell bench press		1 drop set	10-12 (+ as many more as possible)	311	60 secs	
❹ Cable kickback		3	10-12	311	60 secs	
❺ Gym ball oblique crunch		2	10 each side	311	60 secs	n/a
❻ Two point box		2	15 each side	312	60 secs	n/a

Warm down and stretch Ten minutes of gentle cardio plus static stretches (20 seconds each). Focus on chest, triceps, abs, lower back (see p14)

Notes

❶ T press-up

Target: **pecs, shoulders, arms, core**

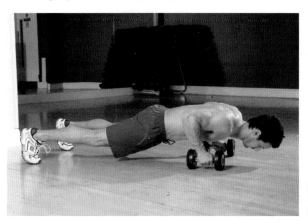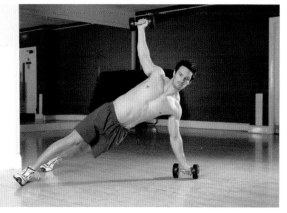

● Grip the dumb-bells with straight wrists, directly below your shoulders.

● Position your feet shoulder width apart, don't let your hips sag.

● Keep your body in a straight line and your elbows tucked into your sides.

● Push up powerfully and twist your

body, rolling onto the sides of your feet while keeping your body straight.

● Raise the dumb-bell overhead with a straight arm, return to the start and repeat on the other side.

❷ Cable pullover

Target: **pecs, lats**

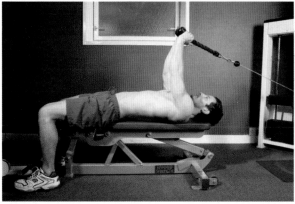

● Support your head and shoulders on a bench and grasp a rope attachment with a hammer grip, over your chest.

● Your feet should be flat on the ground, your core engaged and your body straight from head to knees.

● Keeping a slight bend in your elbows, slowly lower the weight behind your head. Ensure there is tension on the cable throughout

● Pull the weight back to the start using your chest muscles, avoid arching your back to aid the movement.

③ Dumb-bell bench press

Target: **pecs, triceps**

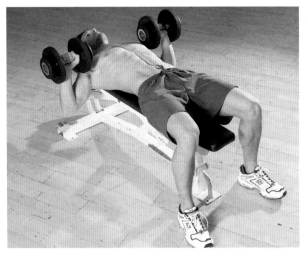
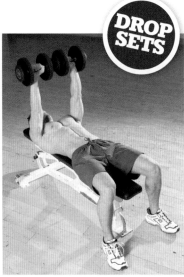

DROP SETS

● Lie on the bench with your knees bent at 90°, your feet flat on the floor and your core braced.

● Hold the dumb-bells at chest level then press them straight up.

● Maintain a natural arch in your back. There should just be enough room to slip a few fingers between your lower back and the bench.

● Lower the weights slowly.

④ Cable kickback

Target: **triceps**

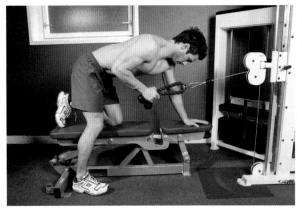
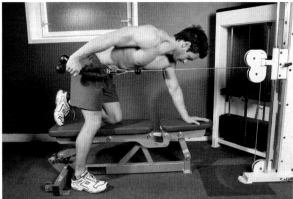

● Rest one knee and one hand on a bench, with your hand directly beneath your shoulder.

● Keep your body horizontal with your upper arm in line with your body, look down so your neck is in line too.

● Grasp a rope attachment to a cable, set just below shoulder height, ensuring there is tension on the cable.

● Press the weight straight back, moving only at your elbow, squeeze your tricep at the top of the move and lower slowly.

⑤ Gym ball oblique crunch

Target: **obliques**

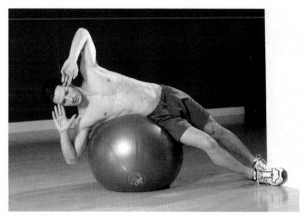 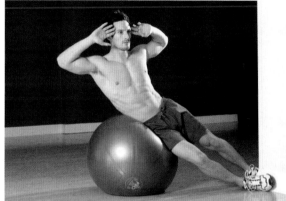

● Lie sideways and curl your body round the ball, jamming your feet against a wall for support.

● Use your side abs to crunch up sideways, hold for a second at the top of the move, and lower under control.

⑥ Two point box

Target: **lower back**

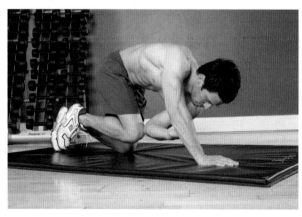 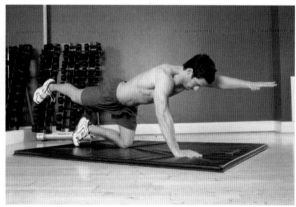

● Kneel on all fours and keep looking down throughout the movement.

● Bring one elbow to meet the opposite knee beneath your stomach before stretching out your arm and leg.

● Your body should form a straight line from foot to fingertip, don't let your hips rotate.

● Hold this position for a count of two, return to the start and repeat on the other side.

WORKOUT C

Your final workout of the week targets your legs, shoulders and core. Using a Smith machine for the squat drop set allows you to change the resistance quickly and means you can perform the move safely even when your quads are fully exhausted.

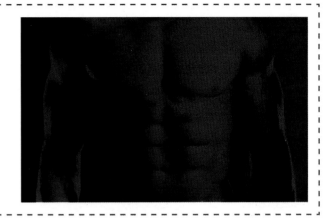

Warm-up Ten minutes of gentle cardio followed by dynamic stretches (see p13)

Exercise		Sets	Reps	Tempo	Rest	Weight
1 Lunge		2	8 each leg	211	60 secs	
2 Push press		3	10-12	31X	60 secs	
3 Smith squat		1 drop set	10-12 (+ as many more as possible)	311	60 secs	
4 Arnold press		3	10-12	311	60 secs	
5 Knee raise		3	8-10	311	60 secs	n/a
6 Gym ball back extension		3	10-12	311	60 secs	n/a

Warm down and stretch Ten minutes of gentle cardio plus static stretches (20 seconds each). Focus on quads, glutes, hams, shoulders, abs, lower back (see p14)

Notes

❶ Lunge

Target: **quads, glutes, hamstrings**

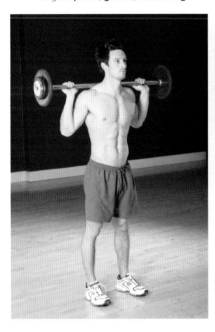 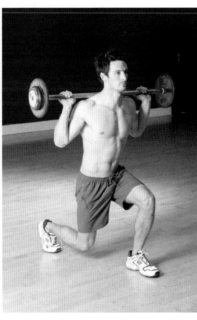

● Stand upright with your core braced and your feet shoulder width apart.

● Rest the bar on the back of your shoulders and keep your elbows back to retract your shoulder blades.

● Take a big step forward, making sure your front knee is over your front foot, sink down until your back knee almost touches the floor.

● Push off your front foot to return to the start.

❷ Push press

Target: **deltoids**

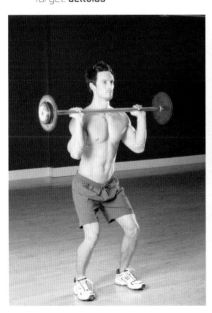 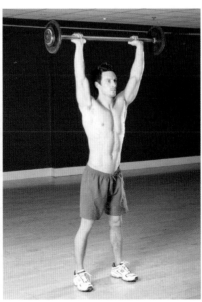

● Stand with your feet shoulder width apart, your body upright, core braced and head looking straight ahead.

● Grip the bar just wider than shoulder width apart and hold it on your upper chest.

● Bend your knees slightly then drive up with your legs and arms at the same time. Press the bar directly overhead without tilting your hips forward. Slowly lower it to the start.

③ Smith squat

Target: **quads, glutes**

DROP SETS

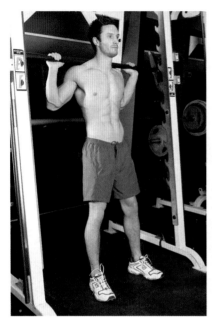
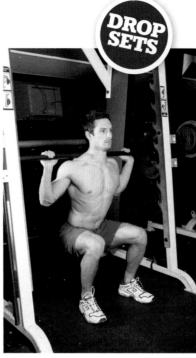

- Place your feet shoulder width apart and slightly in front of your body to put more emphasis on your quads.
- Rest the bar on the back of your shoulders, not your neck, and keep your elbows back.
- Look forward, brace your core and unlock the bar from the rack.
- Maintaining a natural arch in your back, lower until your thighs are parallel to the floor.
- Push back up through your heels.

④ Arnold press

Target: **deltoids**

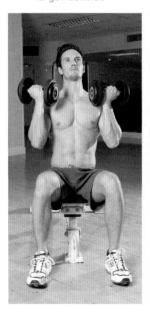
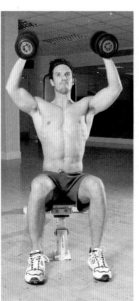
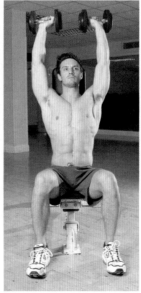

- Sit on a bench with your lower back and shoulders pressed against the pad, keep your feet flat on the floor.
- Hold the dumb-bells at shoulder height, palms facing in and elbows to the front.
- As you press the weights directly overhead rotate your palms so that they finish facing forward.
- Reverse the motion back to the start.

⑤ Knee raise

Target: **lower abdominals**

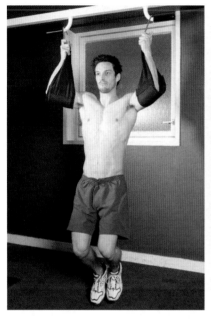
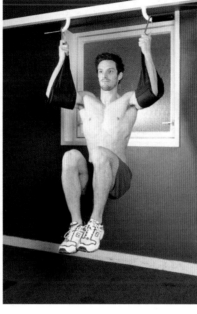

● Hang from a bar using an overhand grip or elbow straps, hold your feet together and try not to swing.

● With your knees bent, use your abs to draw your knees up towards your chest.

● Hold for a second at the top of the move then lower slowly without swinging.

⑥ Gym ball back extension

Target: **lower back**

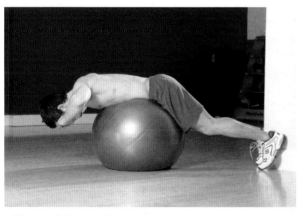
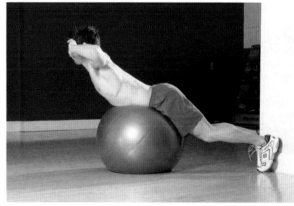

● Wrap your body around the gym ball, jamming your feet against a wall for support.

● Lift your back until your body forms a straight line, being careful not to over-extend.

● Pause for a moment at the top of the exercise before lowering slowly.

WEEK 8

NEGATIVE VIBES

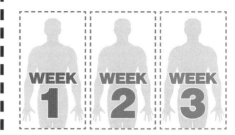

WEEK
1

WEEK
2

WEEK
3

This week you'll try out a new way to stimulate growth in your muscles: 'negatives'.

When you lift a weight your muscle contracts under tension – known as the concentric phase of a lift. By contrast, the eccentric phase is where the muscle lengthens under tension as you lower the weight, and this is what you'll be focussing on this week.

For each 'negative' exercise pick a weight that you would struggle to lift without help and then focus on lowering the weight slowly and under control. If you have a training partner ask him to help you re-set the weight at the start of each rep. If not use whatever safe method you can to lift the weight before doing a slow, controlled negative rep.

Only two exercises per workout are negatives. The others should be performed as normal.

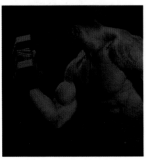

TRAINING PLAN

MON
WORKOUT A
(see p124)

TUE
CARDIO SESSION
200 metre sprints
4 minutes warm-up – level 3
Run 200 metres – level 10
Walk slowly back to start
4 minutes warm down – level 3
x6

WED
WORKOUT B
(see p128)

THU
REST DAY

FRI
WORKOUT C
(see p132)

SAT
CARDIO SESSION
Recovery
Run, swim or cycle at level 6 for 40 minutes, maintaining a steady pace

SUN
REST DAY

MEAL PLAN

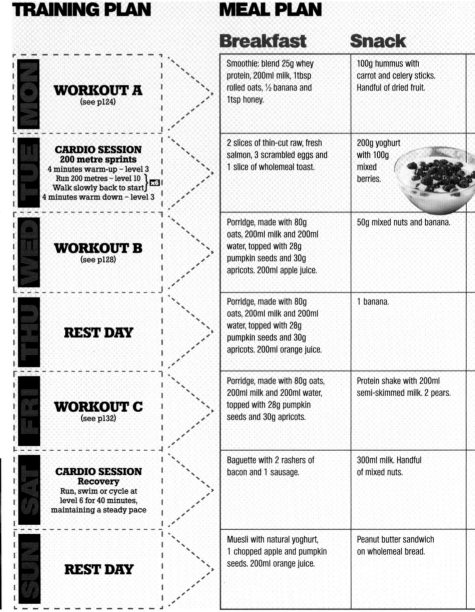

	Breakfast	Snack
MON	Smoothie: blend 25g whey protein, 200ml milk, 1tbsp rolled oats, ½ banana and 1tsp honey.	100g hummus with carrot and celery sticks. Handful of dried fruit.
TUE	2 slices of thin-cut raw, fresh salmon, 3 scrambled eggs and 1 slice of wholemeal toast.	200g yoghurt with 100g mixed berries.
WED	Porridge, made with 80g oats, 200ml milk and 200ml water, topped with 28g pumpkin seeds and 30g apricots. 200ml apple juice.	50g mixed nuts and banana.
THU	Porridge, made with 80g oats, 200ml milk and 200ml water, topped with 28g pumpkin seeds and 30g apricots. 200ml orange juice.	1 banana.
FRI	Porridge, made with 80g oats, 200ml milk and 200ml water, topped with 28g pumpkin seeds and 30g apricots.	Protein shake with 200ml semi-skimmed milk. 2 pears.
SAT	Baguette with 2 rashers of bacon and 1 sausage.	300ml milk. Handful of mixed nuts.
SUN	Muesli with natural yoghurt, 1 chopped apple and pumpkin seeds. 200ml orange juice.	Peanut butter sandwich on wholemeal bread.

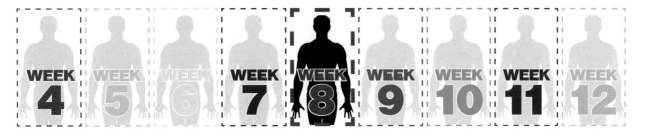
Lunch	Snack	Dinner	Snack	Total
220g roast beef, 3 roast potatoes (halved and cooked in butter), broccoli, cauliflower, asparagus, green beans and butternut squash.	200g yoghurt with 1tsp grated coconut.	150g roast beef with salad (tomato, cucumber, spring onion, grated carrot).	Protein shake: blend 33g casein protein, 150ml milk, 100ml yoghurt, 1tsp honey and a pinch of cinnamon.	**2,990 calories,** 316g protein, 187g carbs, 109g fat
Jacket potato with chilli (300g beef, ½ tin red kidney beans, 1 tin tomatoes and spices).	1tbsp peanut butter. 1 pear. 1 kiwi.	Seafood salad: 1 tin of tuna in brine, 120g cod fillet, 120g prawns, mixed leaf salad, and a sprinkle of grated cheese. 1 banana.	2 chicken wings	**2,890 calories,** 280g protein, 200g carbs, 108g fat
3-egg omelette with chicken and cheese. 50g mixed salad.	Protein shake with 200ml semi-skimmed milk.	Salmon fillet, 250g steamed vegetables (kale, peas and carrots) and 100g boiled new potatoes.	200ml milk.	**3,067 calories,** 152g protein, 258g carbs, 110g fat
3-egg omelette with chicken and cheese. 50g mixed salad.	50g mixed nuts.	Salmon fillet with pak choi, 250g steamed vegetables (kale, peas and carrots) and 100g rice noodles.	Protein shake with 200ml semi-skimmed milk.	**3,036 calories,** 154g protein, 245g carbs, 111g fat
2 wholemeal bagels with smoked salmon and cream cheese.	Peanut butter sandwich on wholemeal bread.	2 turkey fajitas with mixed vegetables and salsa.	75g natural yoghurt with 25g mixed nuts.	**2,950 calories,** 163g protein, 331g carbs, 90g fat
Jacket potato with butter, 1 diced turkey breast, sun-dried tomato and rocket.	125g full-fat cottage cheese. 1 apple. 1 kiwi.	120g lightly fried tuna steak with stir-fried mixed veg (4 varieties).	Protein shake: blend 33g casein protein, 150ml milk, 100ml yoghurt, 1tsp honey and a pinch of cinnamon.	**2,910 calories,** 282g protein, 191g carbs, 113g fat
Grilled chicken with couscous, peppers, courgettes, carrots, onions, pine nuts and apricots.	250ml shop-bought smoothie and cereal bar.	Roast beef with new and roast potatoes, carrots, broccoli, cauliflower, peas and parsnips.	200ml vanilla ice cream.	**2,989 calories,** 149g protein, 297g carbs, 117g fat

WORKOUT A

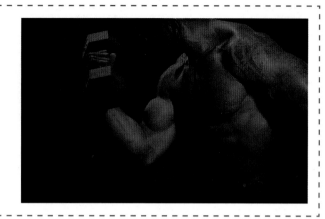

In this workout you'll focus on your back, biceps and core. For the negative exercises use a weight that you would struggle to lift, but which you can control on the eccentric (lowering) portion of the move. Aim to take a full five seconds to lower the weight on the negative exercises.

Warm-up Ten minutes of gentle cardio followed by dynamic stretches (see p13)

Exercise		Sets	Reps	Tempo	Rest	Weight
❶ Bent-over row		3	10-12	311	60 secs	
❷ Negative weighted pull-up		3	8	5--	60 secs	
❸ Bent-over flye		3	10-12	311	60 secs	
❹ Alternating hammer curl with twist		2	8 each arm	311	60 secs	
❺ Negative one-arm preacher curls		3	6 each arm	5--	60 secs	
❻ Medicine ball leg drop		3	10-12	213	60 secs	

Warm down and stretch Ten minutes of gentle cardio plus static stretches (20 seconds each). Focus on quads, hams, lower back, upper back, chest, shoulders (see p14)

Notes

❶ Bent-over row

Target: traps, lats, rhomboids

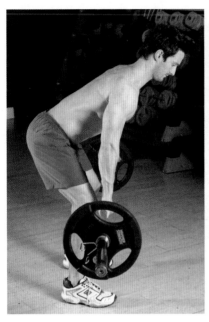 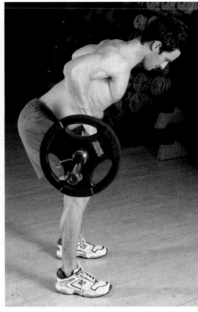

● Start with your core braced, your back straight and your shoulder blades retracted.

● With your knees slightly bent, lean forward from the hips, rather than the waist, keep your back straight.

● Grip the bar just wider than shoulder width apart, letting it hang straight down around knee level.

● Pull the bar up into your sternum, squeezing your shoulder blades together at the top of the move, then lower the bar slowly to the start.

❷ Negative weighted pull-up

Target: lats, traps, rhomboids

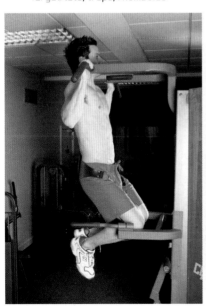 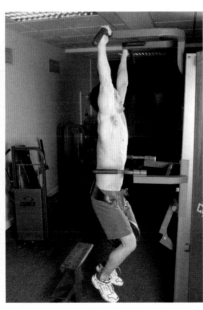

● Hang a weight plate from a belt or hold a dumb-bell between your legs.

● Grip the bar with an overhand grip just wider than shoulder width apart.

● Use a bench or a helper to get your chin over the bar.

● Lower yourself in a slow and controlled manner until your arms are straight.

③ Bent-over flye

Target: **traps, lats, rhomboids**

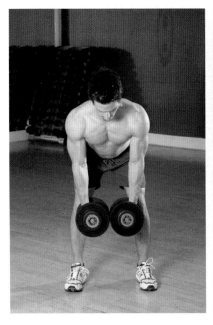
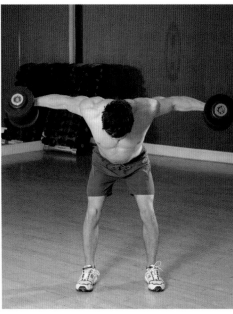

● Start with your core braced, your back straight and your shoulder blades retracted.

● With your knees slightly bent, lean forward from the hips, rather than the waist, keep your back straight.

● Keeping a slight bend in your elbows, raise the weights straight out to the sides without moving your upper body.

● Squeeze your shoulder blades at the top of the movement and lower slowly.

④ Alternating hammer curl with twist

Target: **biceps**

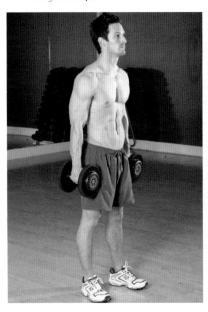
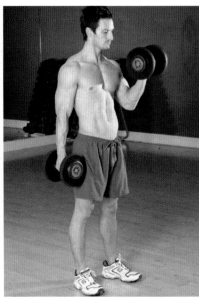

● Stand tall with your shoulders back and your core muscles braced for support.

● Keep your elbows tucked into your sides and, without leaning back, curl up one dumb-bell at a time.

● Turn your wrist out at the top of the move, stop before your forearms are vertical and lower slowly.

⑤ Negative one-arm preacher curls

Target: biceps

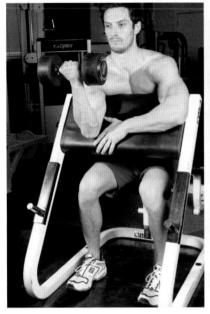 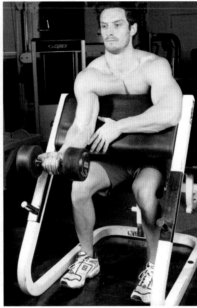

● Sit at a preacher bench with it under your armpits and hold a dumb-bell up with your forearm vertical.

● Press into the pad with your free hand to prevent your body twisting.

● Slowly lower the weight until your arm is almost straight but leave a bend in your elbow.

● Use both hands to re-set the weight.

⑥ Medicine ball leg drop

Target: abdominals, hips, adductors

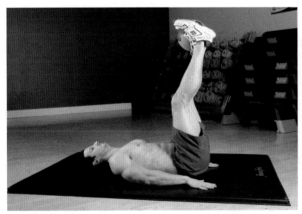 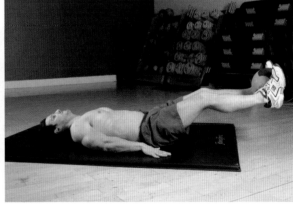

● Lie on your back with your head and shoulders on the floor and your arms flat on the floor for balance.

● Grip a medicine ball between your feet with your legs up in the air.

● Lower as slowly as you can, stopping before you touch the floor, return to the start.

WORKOUT B

Your mid-week workout puts the emphasis on your legs and abs. When you do the negative one-leg Smith squats, use two legs to lift the weight but only one to lower it under control. With the negative cable crunch, use your whole bodyweight to drag the cable down, then only use your abs to control it back up again.

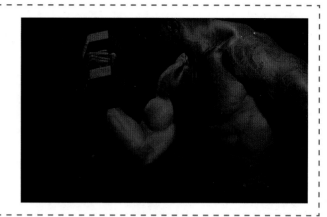

Warm-up Ten minutes of gentle cardio followed by dynamic stretches (see p13)

Exercise		Sets	Reps	Tempo	Rest	Weight
1 High pull		3	10-12	21X	60 secs	
2 Squat		3	10-12	311	60 secs	
3 Negative one-leg Smith squat		3	5 each leg	5--	60 secs	
4 Bicycles		2	30 secs	101	60 secs	n/a
5 Negative cable crunch		3	8	5--	60 secs	
6 Gym ball Russian twist		3	8 each side	101	60 secs	

Warm down and stretch Ten minutes of gentle cardio plus static stretches (20 seconds each). Focus on quads, glutes, hams, traps, abs, lower back (see p14)

Notes

❶ High pull

Target: hamstrings, glutes, calves, back, shoulders

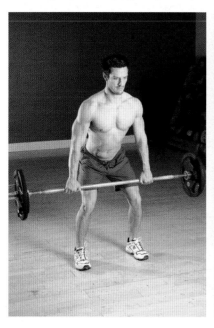 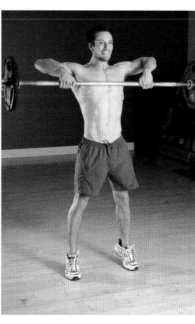

● Stand with your feet shoulder width apart, your back straight, shoulders back and core braced.

● Grip the bar just outside your knees, lean forward from the hips, not the waist, and bend your knees to initiate the move.

● Pull the bar up in front of you powerfully, rising up onto your toes to gain more power and keeping your elbows high.

● Lower the bar in a controlled manner and return to the start.

❷ Squat

Target: quads, glutes, hamstrings

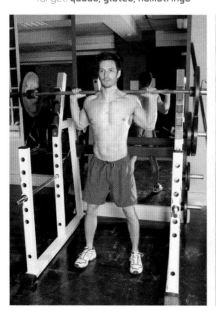 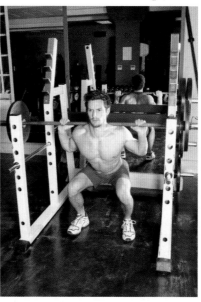

● Stand with your feet shoulder width apart, your toes turned out slightly and your core braced.

● Rest the bar on the back of your shoulders, not your neck, gripping it close to your shoulders.

● Maintain a natural arch in your back, keep your elbows retracted and look forward throughout the movement.

● Lower until your thighs are parallel to the floor, keeping your knees in line with your feet, then push back up through your heels.

❸ Negative one-leg Smith squat

Target: quads, glutes

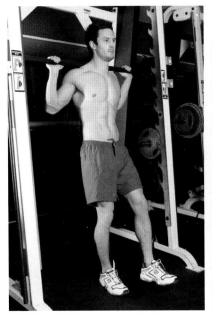 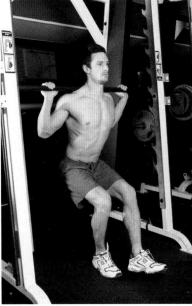

● Place one foot slightly in front of your body to put more emphasis on your quads, keep the other foot off the floor.

● Rest the bar on the back of your shoulders, not your neck, look forward and brace your core.

● Unlock the bar from the rack and lower slowly and under control, as far as feels comfortable.

● Return to the start position using both legs or with help from someone else.

❹ Bicycles

Target: abdominals

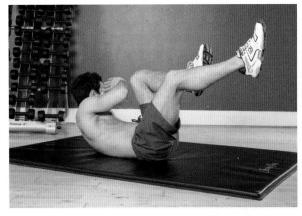 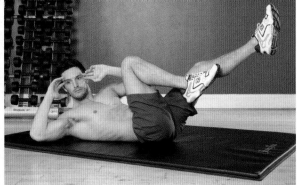

● Start with your fingers by your temples, crunch up to bring your right elbow to your left knee while extending your right leg.

● Twist your torso to the other side as you crunch your left elbow to your right knee and extend your left leg.

● Perform this movement in a quick but controlled manner, being careful not to strain your neck.

⑤ Negative cable crunch

Target: upper abdominals

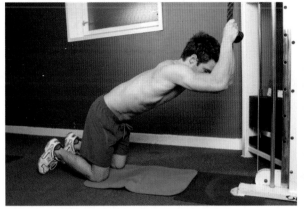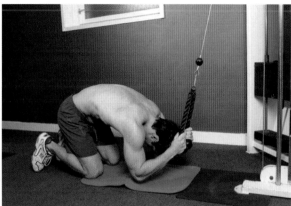

● Start by kneeling on the floor holding a rope handle attached to a high cable, with your chest curled towards your knees.

● Use your whole bodyweight to pull the cable down, then focus on using only your abs to control the movement back up again.

⑥ Gym ball Russian twist

Target: obliques, core

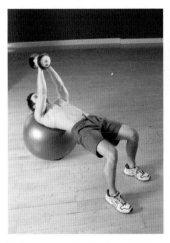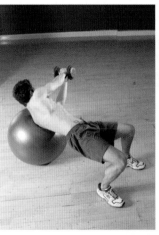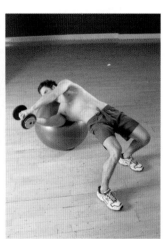

● Rest your head and shoulders on a gym ball with your feet flat and your body in a straight line.

● Hold a dumb-bell straight above your chest, twist your torso over to one side until your arms are parallel to the floor.

● Twist to the other side, looking in the direction of the dumb-bell.

WORKOUT C

The focus will be on your chest and triceps for this workout. For the negative gym ball press-up you can drop to your knees to reset the start position, then aim to take five seconds to lower your body to the ball while minimising the wobble.

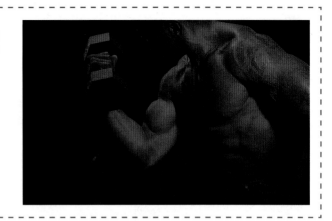

Warm-up Ten minutes of gentle cardio followed by dynamic stretches (see p13)

Exercise		Sets	Reps	Tempo	Rest	Weight
1 Incline bench press		3	10-12	311	60 secs	
2 Negative gym ball press-up		3	6	5--	60 secs	n/a
3 Split squat to one-arm row		2	10-12 each side	311	60 secs	
4 Shoulder press with rotation		3	6 each side	311	60 secs	
5 Seated EZ-bar overhead triceps extension		3	10-12	311	60 secs	
6 Negative unilateral wall press-up		2	6 each arm	5--	60 secs	n/a

Warm down and stretch Ten minutes of gentle cardio plus static stretches (20 seconds each). Focus on chest, triceps, shoulders (see p14)

Notes

❶ Incline bench press

Target: upper pecs, front deltoids, triceps

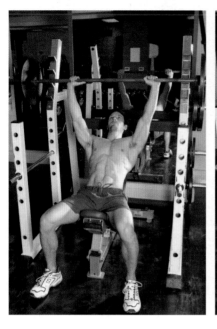 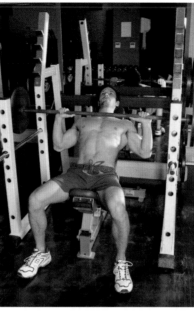

● Lie on a bench set at 30-45° with your feet flat on the floor, your knees bent at 90° and your core braced.

● Grip the bar slightly wider than shoulder width, retract your shoulder blades and lift the bar off the rack, holding it directly over your chest.

● Maintain a natural arch in your back, there should just be enough room to slip a few fingers between your lower back and the bench.

● Lower the bar slowly, keeping your elbows to the sides and press up powerfully.

❷ Negative gym ball press-up

Target: pecs, triceps

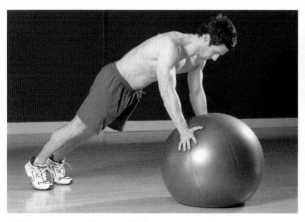 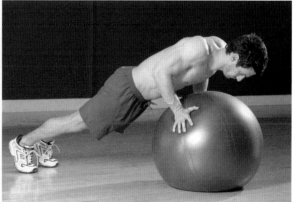

● Brace your core to keep your body in a straight line from head to heels.

● Grip the sides of the ball with your hands roughly in line with your shoulders.

● Slowly lower your body towards the ball, controlling any wobbling.

③ Split squat to one-arm row

Target: legs, back, arms, shoulders, core

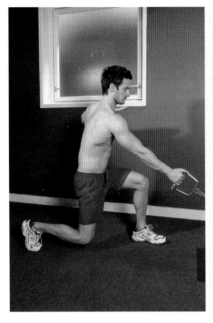
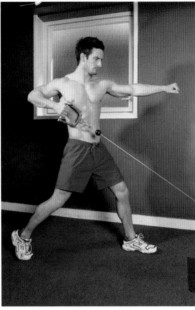

● Start in a lunge position with your left leg forward and your right hand gripping a low cable handle.

● Turn your body towards the cable, keep your head upright and your core braced.

● Without moving your feet, stand up, draw the cable back to your side and retract your shoulder blade while turning your body away from the cable.

④ Shoulder press with rotation

Target: deltoids, core

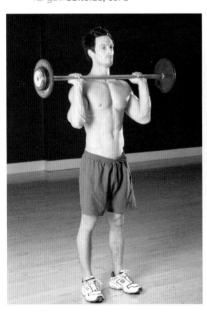
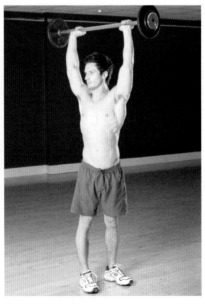

● Stand with your feet shoulder width apart, your body upright, core braced and head looking straight ahead.

● Grip the bar just wider than shoulder width apart and hold it on your upper chest.

● As you press the bar directly overhead rotate your body to the side, using your core muscles to control the motion.

● Slowly return to the start, alternate sides with each rep.

⑤ Seated EZ-bar overhead triceps extension

Target: triceps

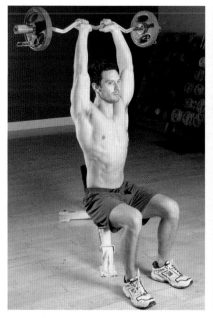 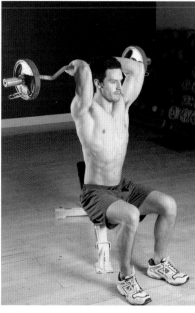

- Sit upright on a bench with your back straight and your feet flat on the floor.

- Hold an EZ-bar directly overhead with your wrists turned in slightly.

- Slowly lower the bar behind your head, keeping the rest of your body still and your upper arms as vertical as possible.

- Press the bar back up powerfully, squeeze your triceps at the top of the move.

⑥ Negative unilateral wall press-up

Target: triceps, chest

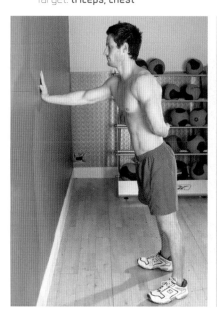 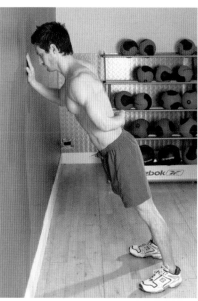

- Stand with your feet slightly wider than shoulder width apart and place one hand on the wall.

- Hold your body in a straight line and slowly lower yourself towards the wall while keeping your elbow close to your side.

- Stand far enough from the wall to make the exercise difficult, and use both hands to press back to the start.

WEEK 9

DOUBLING UP

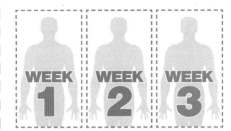

WEEK 1

WEEK 2

WEEK 3

You're into the final four weeks of the *Body Challenge* plan, and now is the time to raise the intensity a bit. For these weeks you'll do full body workouts every time, with the aim of stressing as many muscle fibres as possible. This will flood your body with muscle-building hormones and ramp up your metabolism, which means you'll be burning off fat long after your workout has ended.

This week you'll be doing antagonistic supersets – two exercises done back-to-back with no rest in between. This not only saves you time in the gym but increases your overall work rate to help fire up that muscle-building/fat-burning process. Because the exercises are 'antagonistic' – meaning they work opposing muscle groups – you can rest one muscle while working its opposite.

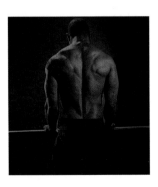

TRAINING PLAN

MON
WORKOUT A
(see p138)

TUE
CARDIO SESSION
Running intervals
4 minutes warm up – level 3
1 minute fast – level 8
1 minute slow – level 4
4 minutes warm down – level 3

WED
WORKOUT B
(see p142)

THU
REST DAY

FRI
WORKOUT C
(see p146)

SAT
CARDIO SESSION
Recovery
Run, swim or cycle at
level 5 for 40 minutes,
maintaining a steady pace

SUN
REST DAY

MEAL PLAN

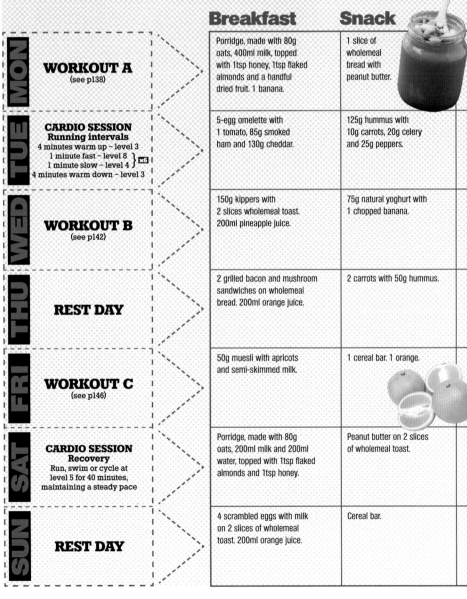

Breakfast	Snack
Porridge, made with 80g oats, 400ml milk, topped with 1tsp honey, 1tsp flaked almonds and a handful dried fruit. 1 banana.	1 slice of wholemeal bread with peanut butter.
5-egg omelette with 1 tomato, 85g smoked ham and 130g cheddar.	125g hummus with 10g carrots, 20g celery and 25g peppers.
150g kippers with 2 slices wholemeal toast. 200ml pineapple juice.	75g natural yoghurt with 1 chopped banana.
2 grilled bacon and mushroom sandwiches on wholemeal bread. 200ml orange juice.	2 carrots with 50g hummus.
50g muesli with apricots and semi-skimmed milk.	1 cereal bar. 1 orange.
Porridge, made with 80g oats, 200ml milk and 200ml water, topped with 1tsp flaked almonds and 1tsp honey.	Peanut butter on 2 slices of wholemeal toast.
4 scrambled eggs with milk on 2 slices of wholemeal toast. 200ml orange juice.	Cereal bar.

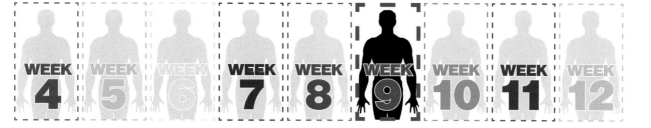

Lunch	Snack	Dinner	Snack	Total
Tuna and mayo baguette. 1 apple.	1 oat cereal bar. 1 banana. 1 orange.	Broccoli tuna pasta bake: 100g pasta, 200g tuna and 85g broccoli florets.	1 slice of toast with peanut butter. Glass of milk.	**3,016 calories,** 95g protein, 227g carbs, 70g fat
1 jacket potato with 200g tuna and ½ tin of sweetcorn.	20g sunflower seeds and 20g pumpkin seeds.	500g lasagne and a green salad with watercress.	Choppped banana.	**3,117 calories,** 132g protein, 190g carbs, 117g fat
Spanish omelette using 4 eggs, potatoes, peppers and onions. Side salad.	Protein shake made with 200ml semi-skimmed milk. 26g pumpkin seeds.	2 Cajun chicken breasts with wholemeal rice and vegetables. 40g 70% cocoa dark organic chocolate.	50g mixed nuts.	**2,975 calories** 130g protein 291g carbs 114g fat
Mixed vegetable 4-egg omelette. Greek salad (feta cheese, olives, sun-dried tomatoes and spinach leaves).	Coconut smoothie: blend 100ml coconut milk, 50ml orange juice, ½ pineapple, 1 banana, 75ml semi-skimmed milk and 1tbsp oats.	Halibut fillet with new potatoes, aubergine, spinach, peas, and carrots. 1 glass of medium white wine.	50g dried fruit and nut mix.	**3,011 calories** 173g protein 269g carbs 176g fat
2 jacket potatoes with tuna and mayonnaise. 250ml cranberry juice.	Peanut butter on 1 slice wholemeal toast.	Turkey stir-fry with peppers, mushrooms, onions and courgettes. 1 pint of lager.	Peanut butter on 1 slice wholemeal toast.	**2,950 calories,** 111g protein, 294g carbs, 67g fat
Steak and cheese wholemeal baguette.	3 celery sticks, 2 carrots and 50g hummus.	2 jacket potatoes with cottage cheese and tuna. Side salad.	200ml semi-skimmed milk.	**3,015 calories,** 117g protein, 302g carbs, 138g fat
Tuna steak with mixed salad (rocket, spinach, peppers, avocado and olives).	Protein shake with 200ml semi-skimmed milk.	2 pork chops with roasted vegetables and sweet potato wedges.	Small bowl of cereal.	**2,990 calories** 163g protein 187g carbs 165g fat

WORKOUT A

In this workout you'll do supersets targeting opposing muscle groups. Do one set of exercise 1a and then immediately do a set of exercise 1b with no rest in between. Rest for 60 seconds before repeating the superset. Follow the same pattern for the other exercises.

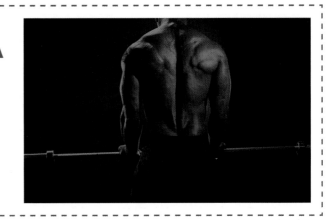

Warm-up Ten minutes of gentle cardio followed by dynamic stretches (see p13)

Exercise		Sets	Reps	Tempo	Rest	Weight
1a	Incline dumb-bell press	3	10-12	311	60 secs	
1b	Lat pull down	3	10-12	311	60 secs	
2a	Squat	3	10-12	311	60 secs	
2b	Romanian deadlift	3	10-12	311	60 secs	
3a	Leg raise	3	8-10	312	60 secs	n/a
3b	Dorsal raise with shoulder rotation	3	10-12	311	60 secs	n/a

Warm down and stretch Ten minutes of gentle cardio plus static stretches (20 seconds each). Focus on chest, lats, triceps, biceps, quads, glutes, hams, abs, lower back (see p14)

Notes

1a Incline dumb-bell press

Target: **upper pecs, front deltoids, triceps**

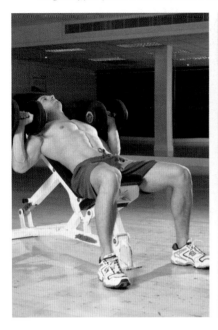
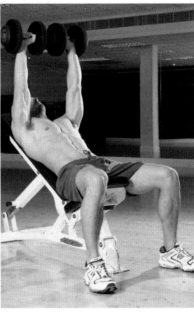

● Lie on a bench set at 30-45° with your feet flat on the floor, your knees bent at 90° and your core braced.

● Hold the dumb-bells at shoulder height, with your palms facing forward, retract your shoulder blades and press the weights straight up.

● Maintain a natural arch in your back, there should just be enough room to slip a few fingers between your lower back and the bench.

1b Lat pull down

Target: **lats, traps, rhomboids**

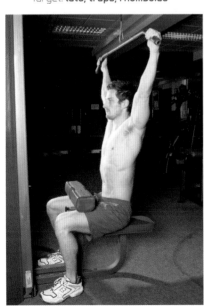
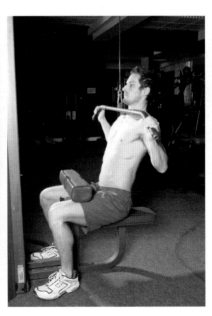

● With your thighs secured snugly under the pad, keep your torso upright and take a wide grip on the bar.

● Without leaning back too far, pull the bar down to your upper chest, and squeeze your lats.

● Allow the bar to raise up to the start slowly and under control.

2a Squat

Target: quads, glutes, hamstrings

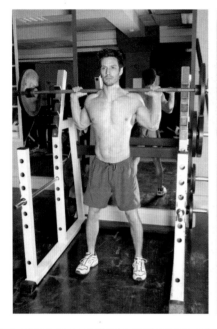 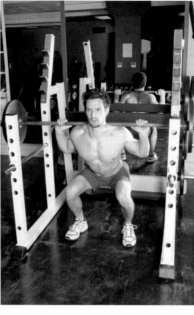

- Stand with your feet shoulder width apart, your toes turned out slightly and your core braced.
- Rest the bar on the back of your shoulders, not your neck, gripping it close to your shoulders.
- Maintain a natural arch in your back, keep your elbows retracted and look forward throughout the movement.
- Lower until your thighs are parallel to the floor, keeping your knees in line with your feet, then push back up through your heels.

2b Romanian deadlift

Target: hamstrings

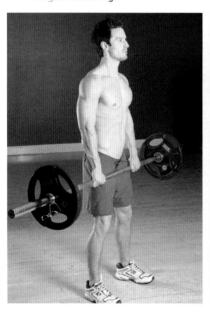 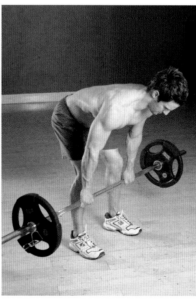

- Stand with your feet shoulder width apart and your head up.
- Keep looking forward, with your shoulders back and core braced.
- Grip the bar just outside your hips and initiate the move by leaning forward from the hips rather than the waist.
- Allow a slight bend in your knees, keep your back straight and push your hips back as the bar travels down your shins.
- Lower the bar until you feel a good stretch in your hamstrings then reverse the movement to the start.

3a **Leg raise**

Target: **Lower abdominals**

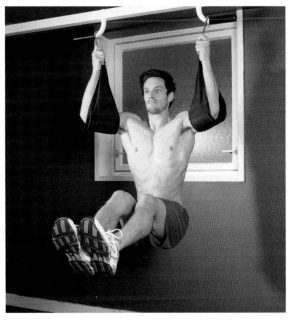

● Hang from a bar using an overhand grip or elbow straps, hold your feet together and try not to swing.

● Keep your legs as straight as you can, use your abs to draw your legs up.

● Hold for a second at the top of the move then lower slowly without swinging.

3b **Dorsal raise with shoulder rotation**

Target: **lower back, upper back**

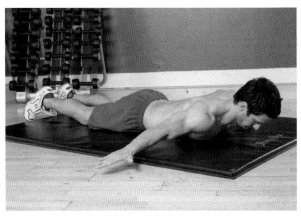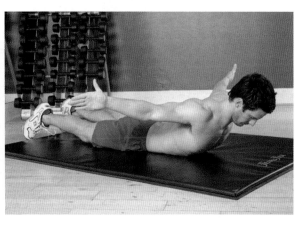

● Lie face down on a mat with your arms held off the floor, out to your sides, palms facing down.

● Use your lower-back muscles to lift your chest off the mat.

● Squeeze your shoulder blades together and twist your hands back so your thumbs point up, hold for a second then reverse to the start.

WORKOUT B

Repeat the superset process as laid out in the previous workout. You'll work all the muscles of your upper body with a series of compound moves that will stimulate maximum muscle growth.

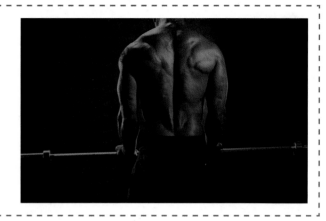

Warm-up Ten minutes of gentle cardio followed by dynamic stretches (see p13)

Exercise		Sets	Reps	Tempo	Rest	Weight
1a Bench press		3	10-12	311	60 secs	
1b Bent-over row		3	10-12	311	60 secs	
2a Dip		3	10-12	211	60 secs	n/a
2b High pull		3	10-12	21X	60 secs	
3a Gym ball passing jackknife		3	10-12	212	60 secs	n/a
3b Good morning		3	10-12	311	60 secs	

Warm down and stretch Ten minutes of gentle cardio plus static stretches (20 seconds each). Focus on chest, traps, triceps, abs, lower back (see p14)

Notes

1a Bench press

Target: pecs, triceps

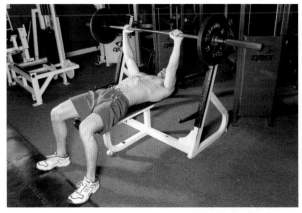 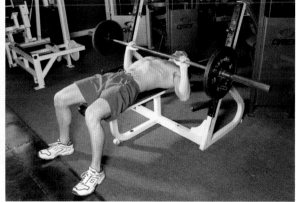

● Lie on the bench with your knees bent at 90°, your feet flat on the floor and your core braced.

● Grip the bar wider than shoulder width, retract your shoulder blades and lift the bar off the rack, holding it directly over your chest.

● Maintain a natural arch in your back. There should be just enough room to slip a few fingers between your lower back and the bench.

● Lower the bar to your chest slowly and press up powerfully.

1b Bent-over row

Target: traps, lats, rhomboids

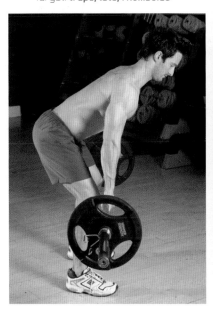 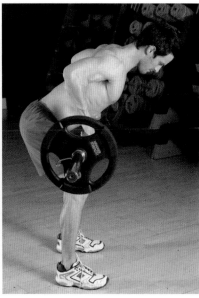

● Start with your core braced, your back straight and your shoulder blades retracted.

● With your knees slightly bent, lean forward from the hips, rather than the waist, keep your back straight.

● Grip the bar just wider than shoulder width apart, letting it hang straight down around knee level.

● Pull the bar up into your sternum, squeezing your shoulder blades together at the top of the move, then lower the bar slowly to the start.

2a Dip

Target: **triceps, chest**

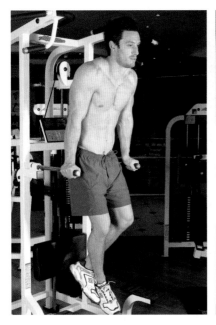 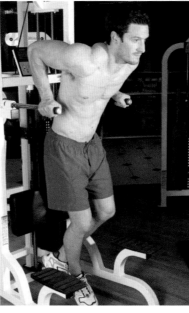

- Grip parallel bars just wider than hip width and keep your body straight.
- Keeping your elbows pointing back, lower yourself slowly as far as is comfortable.
- Push back up powerfully, don't swing your legs for momentum.

2b High pull

Target: **hamstrings, glutes, calves, back, shoulders**

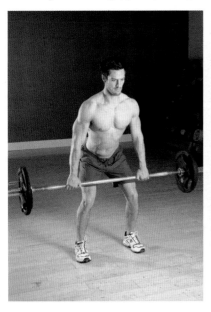 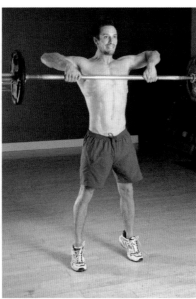

- Stand with your feet shoulder width apart, your back straight, shoulders back and core braced.
- Grip the bar just outside your knees, lean forward from the hips, not the waist, and bend your knees to initiate the move.
- Pull the bar up in front of you powerfully, rising up onto your toes to gain more power and keeping your elbows high.
- Lower the bar in a controlled manner and return to the start.

3a Gym ball passing jackknife

Target: upper and lower abdominals

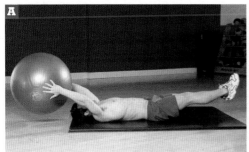

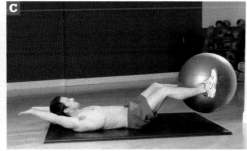

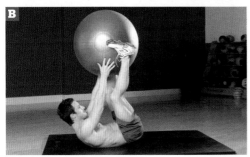

- Start with your body flat on the floor and your feet together, resting on top of the ball.
- Brace your core and raise your hips until your body forms a straight line from your shoulders to your heels.
- Roll the ball towards your backside with your heels, raising your hips to keep your body straight.
- Pause at the top of the movement and slowly return to the start.

3b Good morning

Target: lower back, hamstrings

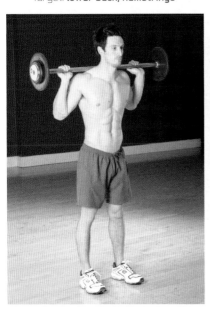

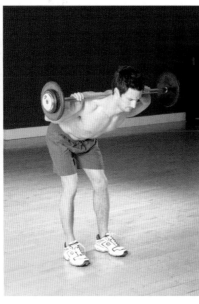

- Stand with your feet shoulder width apart, body upright, core braced and shoulders back.
- Rest the bar across the back of your shoulders, not your neck, with your hands just outside your shoulders.
- Bend forward from the hips not the waist, keeping a natural arch in your back and a slight bend in your knees.
- Push your hips back to maintain balance and lean as far forward as the stretch in your hamstrings will allow.
- Don't let your upper body move beyond horizontal to the floor, reverse the move to the start.

WORKOUT C

In the last of your superset workouts you'll target your upper and lower body with opposing movements: pushing and pulling; squatting and bending; flexion and extension.

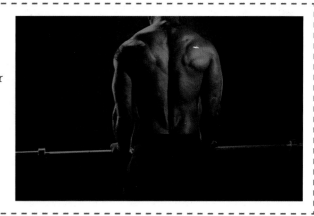

Warm-up Ten minutes of gentle cardio followed by dynamic stretches (see p13)

Exercise		Sets	Reps	Tempo	Rest	Weight
1a Pull-up		3	6-10	311	60 secs	n/a
1b Shoulder press		3	10-12	311	60 secs	
2a Sumo squat		3	10-12	311	60 secs	
2b Gym ball leg curl		3	12-15	311	60 secs	n/a
3a EZ-bar biceps curl		3	10-12	311	60 secs	
3b Seated EZ-bar overhead triceps extension		3	10-12	311	60 secs	

Warm down and stretch Ten minutes of gentle cardio plus static stretches (20 seconds each). Focus on lats, shoulders, quads, hams, adductors, hip flexors, biceps, triceps (see p14)

Notes

1a Pull-up

Target: **lats, traps, rhomboids**

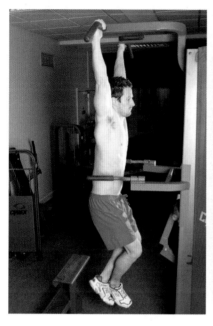
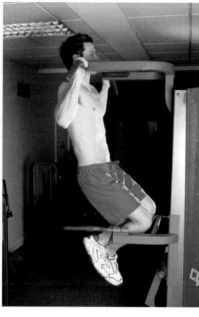

● Grip the bar with an overhand grip just wider than shoulder width apart.

● Extend your arms fully, letting your body hang straight down without swinging.

● Pull up until your chin is over the bar, squeezing your lats as you do.

● Lower slowly without swinging.

1b Shoulder press

Target: **deltoids**

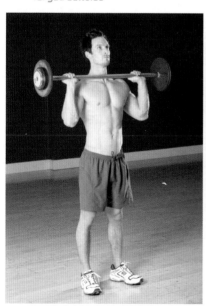
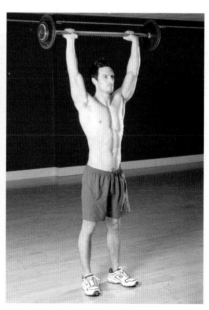

● Stand with your feet shoulder width apart, your body upright, core braced and head looking straight ahead.

● Grip the bar just wider than shoulder width apart and hold it on your upper chest.

● Press the bar directly overhead without tilting your hips forward, slowly lower it to the start.

2a Sumo squat

Target: **quads**

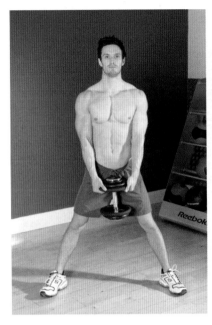
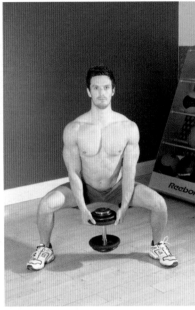

● Take a wide stance with your toes pointing out, grip a dumb-bell by the end.

● Keep looking forward, brace your core and keep your back upright.

● Squat down, keeping your knees in line with your toes, until your thighs are parallel to the floor.

● Press back up powerfully.

2b Gym ball leg curl

Target: **hamstrings**

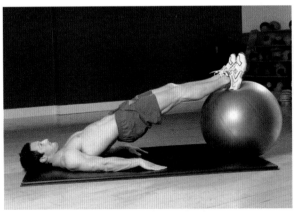
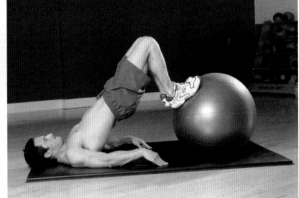

● Rest your head and shoulders on the floor and your heels on top of the ball, your body should be straight from shoulders to heels.

● Raise your hips and drag the ball towards your backside with your heels, keeping your body straight.

● Pause at the top of the movement and return slowly to the start.

3a EZ-bar biceps curl

Target: **biceps**

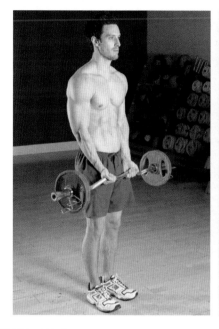
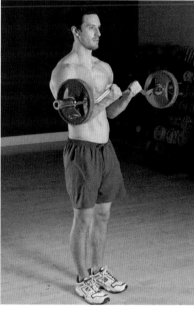

● Stand tall with your shoulders back and your core muscles braced for support.

● Keep your elbows tucked into your sides and grip the EZ-bar with your hands turned inwards slightly.

● Lift the bar without rocking back and forth for momentum, stop before your forearms are vertical and lower slowly.

3b Seated EZ-bar overhead triceps extension

Target: **triceps**

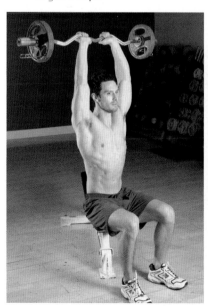
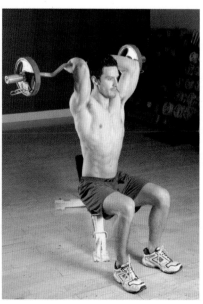

● Sit upright on a bench with your back straight and your feet flat on the floor.

● Hold an EZ-bar directly overhead with your wrists turned in slightly.

● Slowly lower the bar behind your head, keeping the rest of your body still and your upper arms as vertical as possible.

● Press the bar back up powerfully, squeeze your triceps at the top of the move.

WEEK 10
OLYMPIAN HEIGHTS

WEEK 1

WEEK 2

WEEK 3

This week you'll continue with the all-body workouts, with the focus on hitting as many muscle groups as you can. And there aren't many better ways of doing that than with Olympic lifts. These exercises require you to lift a heavy bar to above your head using a series of dynamic moves. Because they are done at speed and use so many muscle groups, their effect is to stimulate a huge surge of testosterone, which is vital in the muscle-building process.

Each workout begins with one of these Olympic-style lifts, and you should note the 'X' on the tempo guides. This means you should perform the moves explosively, but under control.

Also note that for many of the exercises this week the rep count has come down to 8-10, so be sure to adjust the resistance you use accordingly.

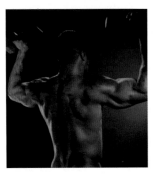

TRAINING PLAN

MON

WORKOUT A
(see p152)

TUE

CARDIO SESSION
Running hill intervals
Run up a steep hill or long set of steps for 1 minute. Jog down again slowly. Repeat 7 times. Afterwards run at level 3 for 5 minutes to warm down.

WED

WORKOUT B
(see p156)

THU

REST DAY

FRI

WORKOUT C
(see p160)

SAT

CARDIO SESSION
Recovery
Run, swim or cycle at level 5 for 40 minutes, maintaining a steady pace

SUN

REST DAY

MEAL PLAN

Breakfast	Snack
2 rashers bacon, 2 poached eggs, 1 sausage and 2 slices wholemeal toast.	125g full-fat cottage cheese. 1 apple.
4 scrambled eggs with milk on 2 slices wholemeal toast. 200ml orange juice.	Cereal bar.
150g lightly fried calf's liver, ½ tin of low-sugar baked beans and 1 slice wholemeal toast.	100g hummus with carrot and celery sticks.
Scramble 2 egg yolks and 5 whites. Serve on 2 slices wholemeal toast with tomato ketchup.	1 granola bar with 110g blueberries, 1tbsp brown sugar, 225g low-fat natural yoghurt, 1 apple, 140ml semi-skimmed milk.
Porridge, made with 80g oats, 200ml milk and 200ml water, topped with 28g pumpkin seeds and 30g apricots.	Protein shake with 200ml semi-skimmed milk. 1 pear.
Porridge, made with 80g oats, 200ml milk and 200ml water, topped with 28g pumpkin seeds and 30g apricots. 200ml orange juice.	1 banana.
Mix 50g rolled oats and 6 egg whites with water into a paste. Cook like a pancake in a non-stick pan. Serve with sugar-free fruit spread.	Place 1 slice ham, cheese and 1 pineapple ring on top of 1 slice wholemeal toast, season with curry powder and pepper, and grill until the cheese is melted. Glass of orange juice.

Lunch	Snack	Dinner	Snack	Total
2 burgers made with 250g minced beef, 1 egg. Mixed salad.	1 pitta with 15g goat's cheese, 15g cheddar and 15g red Leicester. 1 grilled tomato.	¼ roast chicken with mixed grilled vegetables.	Protein shake: blend 33g casein protein, 150ml milk, 100ml yoghurt, 1tsp honey and a pinch of cinnamon. 35g mixed nuts.	**3,160 calories,** 309g protein, 148g carbs, 148g fat
Tuna steak with mixed salad (rocket, spinach, peppers, avocado and olives).	1 slice wholemeal toast and peanut butter.	2 pork chops with roasted vegetables and sweet potato wedges.	Protein shake with 200ml semi-skimmed milk.	**2,990 calories,** 163g protein, 187g carbs, 165g fat
½ roast chicken with salad (beetroot, radish, romaine lettuce and a few seeds).	50g mixed nuts. 1 pear. 1 banana.	250g fillet steak with mixed grilled vegetables.	300ml milk. 1 apple.	**2,947 calories,** 298g protein, 175g carbs, 118g fat
1 wholemeal bagel with 1tbsp peanut butter and 225g cottage cheese.	Raisin and almond snack bar. 2 oranges	Sprinkle a dash of pepper, a squeeze of lemon and 1tbsp grated Parmesan over 115g rainbow trout. Place in tinfoil with a chopped onion and cook for 20-30 minutes. Stir-fry 200g broccoli florets with a clove of crushed garlic. Serve with 50g brown rice.	150g strawberries.	**2,848 calories** 163g protein 401g carbs 77g fat
2 wholemeal bagels with smoked salmon and cream cheese.	Peanut butter sandwich on wholemeal bread. 1 apple.	2 turkey fajitas with mixed vegetables and salsa.	75g natural yoghurt with 25g mixed nuts.	**2,950 calories,** 163g protein, 331g carbs, 90g fat
3-egg omelette with chicken and cheese. 50g mixed salad.	50g mixed nuts.	Salmon fillet, 250g steamed vegetables (kale, peas and carrots) and baked sweet potato.	Protein shake with 200ml semi-skimmed milk.	**3,067 calories,** 152g protein, 258g carbs, 110g fat
Stuff 1 wholemeal tortilla wrap with 1 grilled chicken breast and grilled vegetables.	A handful of prawns with salad leaves.	Sushi made with 100g brown rice, seaweed and salad.	100g cottage cheese with blueberries. 2 kiwi fruits.	**2,950 calories,** 180g protein, 310g carbs, 110g fat

WORKOUT A

The clean and press in this workout should be performed with dynamic movements that can put a lot of strain on your body, so be sure to warm up thoroughly before you start. Practise the movement with an empty bar before adding the appropriate weight.

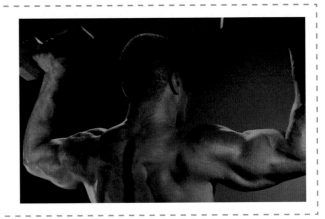

Warm-up Ten minutes of gentle cardio followed by dynamic stretches (see p13)

Exercise		Sets	Reps	Tempo	Rest	Weight
1 Clean and press		3	8-10	31X	60 secs	
2 Cable row		3	8-10	311	60 secs	
3 Lunge		2	8 each leg	211	60 secs	
4 Dumb-bell bench press		3	8-10	311	60 secs	
5 Front/lateral raise		3	10-12	311	60 secs	
6 Medicine ball leg drop		3	10-12	312	60 secs	

Warm down and stretch Ten minutes of gentle cardio plus static stretches (20 seconds each). Focus on traps, shoulders, quads, hams, adductors, chest, triceps, abs (see p14)

Notes

❶ Clean and press

Target: **hamstrings, glutes, calves, back, shoulders**

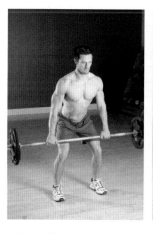 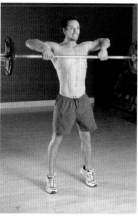 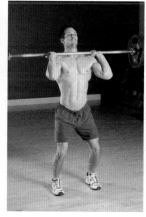 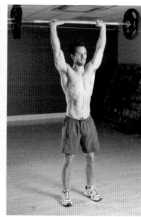

● Stand with your feet shoulder width apart, your back straight, shoulders back and core braced.

● Grip the bar just outside your knees, lean forward from the hips, not the waist, and bend your knees to initiate the move.

● Pull the bar up in front of you powerfully, rising up onto your toes to gain more power and keeping your elbows high.

● Bend your knees to duck under the bar at its highest point, flipping it onto your fingers and catching it on top of your chest.

● Drive up from your knees and press the bar directly overhead.

● Lower the bar in a controlled manner and return to the start.

❷ Cable row

Target: **mid traps, lats, rhomboids**

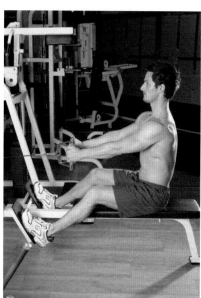 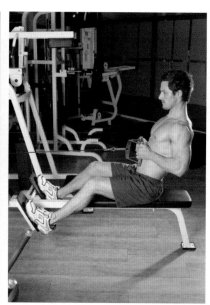

● Sit with a slight bend in your knees, your back straight, shoulder blades retracted and head looking forward.

● Take a neutral grip on the bar and ensure that there is tension in the cable.

● Keeping upper body movement to a minimum, pull the bar into your sternum and squeeze your shoulder blades together.

● Return in a slow and controlled manner.

③ Lunge

Target: quads, hamstrings

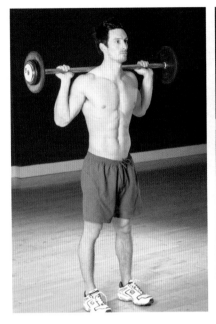
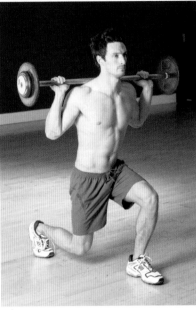

- Stand upright with your core braced and your feet shoulder width apart.

- Rest the bar on the back of your shoulders and keep your elbows back to retract your shoulder blades.

- Take a big step forward, making sure your front knee is over your front foot, sink down until your back knee almost touches the floor.

- Push off your front foot to return to the start.

④ Dumb-bell bench press

Target: pecs, triceps

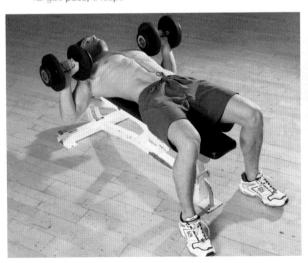
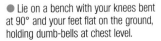
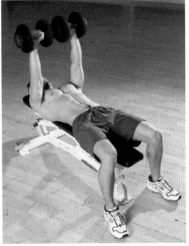

- Lie on a bench with your knees bent at 90° and your feet flat on the ground, holding dumb-bells at chest level.

- Brace your core muscles and, without arching your back, press the weights straight up, then slowly lower.

⑤ **Front/lateral raise**

Target: **front and middle deltoids**

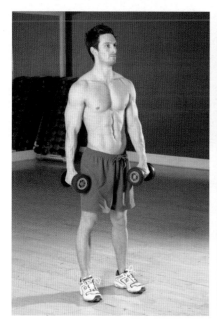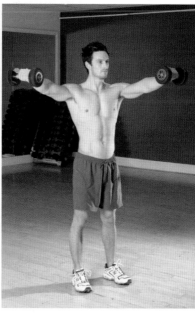

● Stand with your feet shoulder width apart, body upright and core braced.

● Using light dumb-bells hold one by your side and the other in front of you, palms facing in.

● Keeping your arms straight, lift to the side and the front simultaneously without swinging your body for momentum.

● Stop lifting at shoulder height and hold for a moment before lowering slowly and alternating sides.

⑥ **Medicine ball leg drop**

Target: **abdominals, hips, adductors**

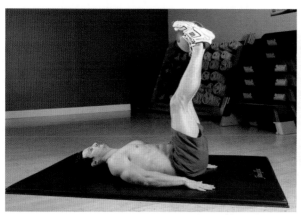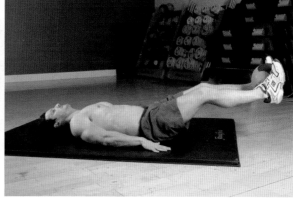

● Lie on your back with your head and shoulders on the floor and your arms flat on the floor for balance.

● Grip a medicine ball between your feet with your legs up in the air.

● Lower as slowly as you can, stopping before you touch the floor, then return to the start.

WORKOUT B

The snatch is one of the hardest moves to get right. It requires good core stability and flexibility in the shoulder, knee and hip joints. Warm up these joints thoroughly and practise the move with light weights first. Only add the resistance gradually until you find the weight you can manage.

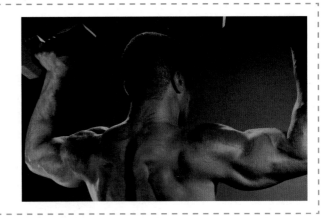

Warm-up Ten minutes of gentle cardio followed by dynamic stretches (see p13)

Exercise		Sets	Reps	Tempo	Rest	Weight
① Snatch		3	8-10	31X	60 secs	
② Cable lateral lunge		3	8 each side	311	60 secs	
③ Chin-up		3	6-10	311	60 secs	n/a
④ Seated dumb-bell shoulder press		3	8-10	311	60 secs	
⑤ Weighted bench dip		3	8-10	211	60 secs	n/a
⑥ Seated Russian twist		3	8 each side	101	60 secs	

Warm down and stretch Ten minutes of gentle cardio plus static stretches (20 seconds each). Focus on traps, shoulders, quads, hams, glutes, chest, lats, triceps, lower back (see p14)

Notes

❶ Snatch

Target: hamstrings, glutes, calves, back, shoulders

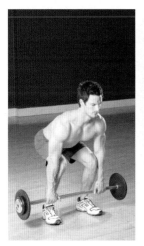 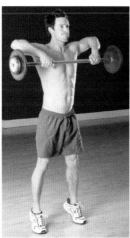 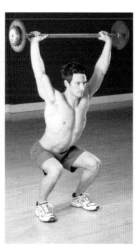 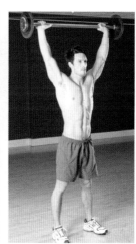

● Start in a deadlift position with the bar off the floor.

● Ensure you keep your back flat, your shoulders retracted and your core braced.

● Lift the bar powerfully, rising up onto your toes to gain more power and keeping your elbows high.

● Duck beneath the bar to 'catch' it with straight arms, maintaining

a natural arch in your back.

● Stand up straight with the bar overhead, lower the bar to the start in a controlled manner.

❷ Cable lateral lunge

Target: adductors, quads, glutes

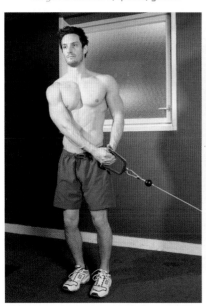 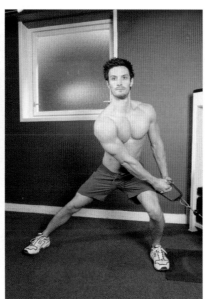

● Stand side-on to a low cable with your torso upright.

● Step sideways towards the cable, lowering onto the leading leg while keeping your knee in line with your foot.

● Stay facing forward, keeping your torso upright, and push back up to your starting position.

③ Chin-up

Target: biceps, lats

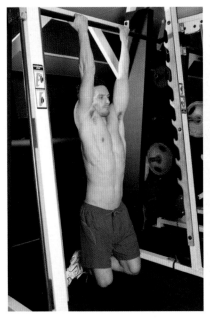
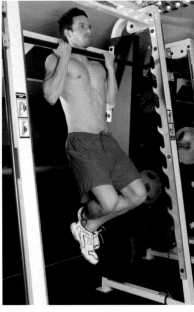

● Grasp the bar with an underhand grip, hands shoulder width apart.

● Lower until your arms are fully extended, cross your legs behind you and try not to swing.

● Pull up until your chin is over the bar and squeeze your biceps hard at the top of the move.

● Lower slowly to the start without swinging.

④ Seated dumb-bell shoulder press

Target: deltoids

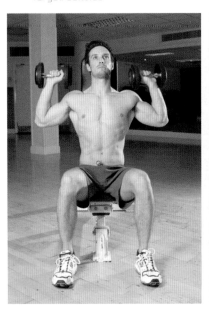
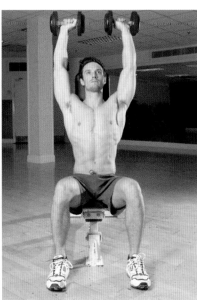

● Sit on a bench with your lower back and shoulders pressed against the pad.

● Keeping your feet flat on the floor, hold the dumb-bells at shoulder height with your elbows out to the sides.

● Press the weights directly overhead but don't let them touch at the top. Lower slowly.

● Keep your core braced throughout and don't arch your back.

⑤ Weighted bench dip

Target: **triceps**

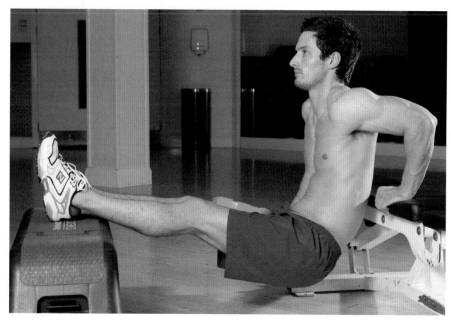

● Grip the edge of the bench with your hands facing forward.

● Place your feet on a bench of the same height with your legs straight, your feet together and a weight plate on your lap.

● Keeping your back upright, lower your body straight down, keeping your elbows pointing back, then press back up powerfully.

⑥ Seated Russian twist

Target: **obliques, core**

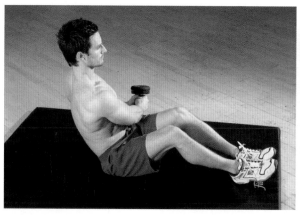 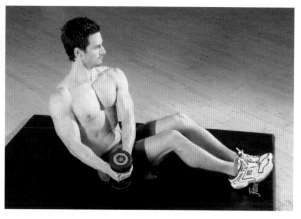

● Sit with your body held at around 45° to the floor, look forward and keep your back straight.

● Bend your knees at 45° and hold a dumb-bell in both hands at arm's length.

● Twist your torso to one side, then to the other, using your abs to control the movement of the dumb-bell.

● Maintain the angle of your upper body to the floor and stay looking forward throughout.

WORKOUT C

The clean and jerk is perhaps the most classic Olympic lift, offering a full-body workout in itself. Once again, take the time to warm up properly and practise the exercise before attempting it with a loaded bar. Aim to keep your core muscles activated during each part of the move.

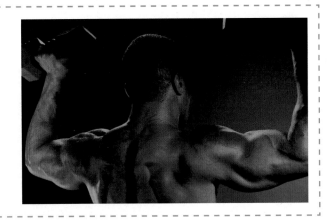

Warm-up Ten minutes of gentle cardio followed by dynamic stretches (see p13)

Exercise		Sets	Reps	Tempo	Rest	Weight
1 Clean and jerk		3	8-10	31X	60 secs	
2 Dumb-bell pullover		3	8-10	311	60 secs	
3 Front squat		3	8-10	311	60 secs	
4 Shrug		3	8-10	211	60 secs	
5 EZ-bar preacher curl		3	8-10	311	60 secs	
6 Modified V-sit		3	10-12	211	60 secs	n/a

Warm down and stretch Ten minutes of gentle cardio plus static stretches (20 seconds each). Focus on traps, shoulders, quads, hams, glutes, lats, triceps, biceps, abs (see p14)

Notes

① Clean and jerk

Target: hamstrings, glutes, calves, back, shoulders

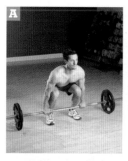 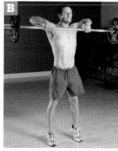 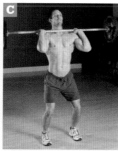

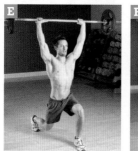 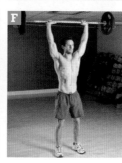

- Start in a deadlift position, ensure you keep your back flat, your shoulders retracted and your core braced.
- Lift the bar powerfully, rising up onto your toes to gain more power and keeping your elbows high.
- Bend your knees to duck under the bar at its highest point, flipping it onto your fingers and catching it on top of your chest.
- Stand up straight and steady yourself then drop into a lunge and press the bar overhead simultaneously.
- Stand up straight then lower the bar in a controlled manner, return to the start.

② Dumb-bell pullover

Target: pecs, lats

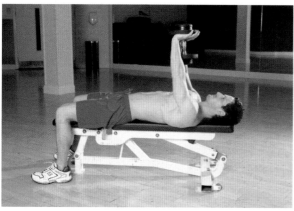 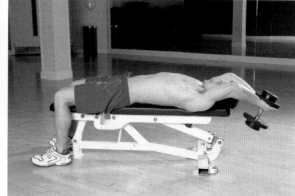

- Support your head and shoulders on a bench with a dumb-bell in both hands over your chest.
- Your feet should be flat on the ground, your core engaged and your body straight from head to knees.

- Keeping a slight bend in your elbows, slowly lower the weight behind your head.
- Pull the weight back to the start using your chest muscles, avoid arching your back to aid the movement.

③ **Front squat**

Target: quads, glutes

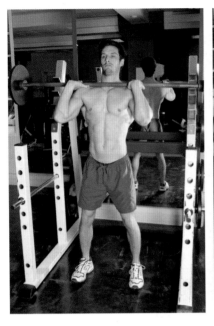
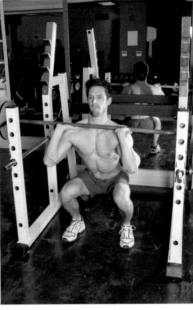

● Stand with your feet shoulder width apart, your toes turned out slightly and your core braced.

● Rest the bar on the front of your shoulders, gripping it with your fingertips.

● Keep your elbows high, maintain a natural arch in your back and look forward throughout the movement.

● Lower until your thighs are parallel to the floor, keeping your knees in line with your feet, then push back up through your heels.

④ **Shrug**

Target: upper traps

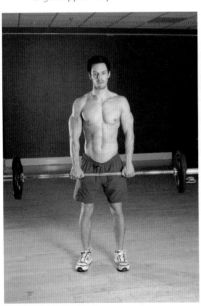
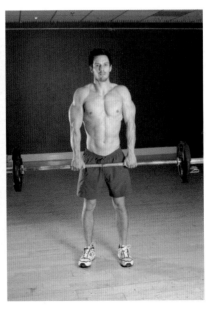

● Stand upright with your shoulders back, grip the bar just outside your thighs.

● Without letting your elbows bend, raise your shoulders straight up and hold for 1-2 seconds.

⑤ EZ-bar preacher curl

Target: **biceps**

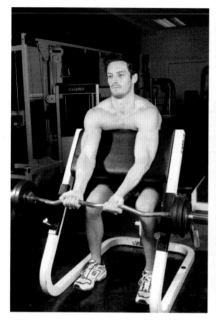
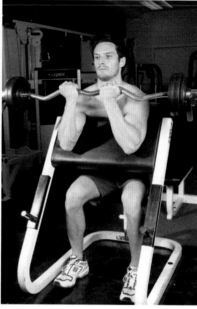

● Sit at a preacher bench with it under your armpits and your elbows resting on the pad.

● Hold an EZ-bar with your wrists turned inwards slightly, keeping a slight bend in your elbows at the lowest point.

● Without lifting your elbows off the pad, curl the bar up towards your shoulders.

● Squeeze your biceps at the top of the move, then slowly lower the weight.

⑥ Modified V-sit

Target: **upper and lower abdominals**

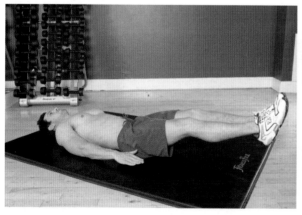
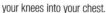
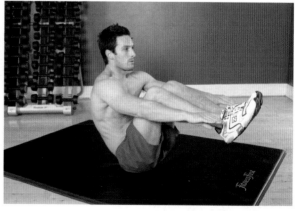

● Lie on a mat with your arms by your sides, your feet raised and your legs straight.

● Sit up, bringing your lower back off the mat, and draw your knees into your chest.

● Balance on your bum at the top of the move before reversing the move in a controlled manner.

WEEK 11
CLUSTER POWER

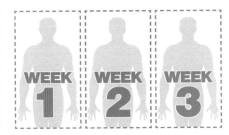

WEEK **1** WEEK **2** WEEK **3**

Only two weeks to go and there's no drop off just yet. This week you'll use the power of cluster sets to fire up your muscles. This is how it works. Most people go to the gym and knock out three sets of ten reps, resting for a minute or so, before moving on to the next exercise. With clusters, you take the same weight you would normally use, but only do four reps, rest for ten seconds and do another four reps. Five of these mini sets makes one cluster. Do three clusters and you'll have done double your normal number of reps without hitting failure.

Of course, this is an intense way of training so it's not for every exercise or even every workout. You'll do one cluster per workout for this week only. All the other exercises should be done as normal.

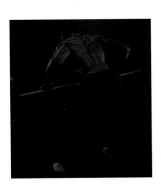

TRAINING PLAN

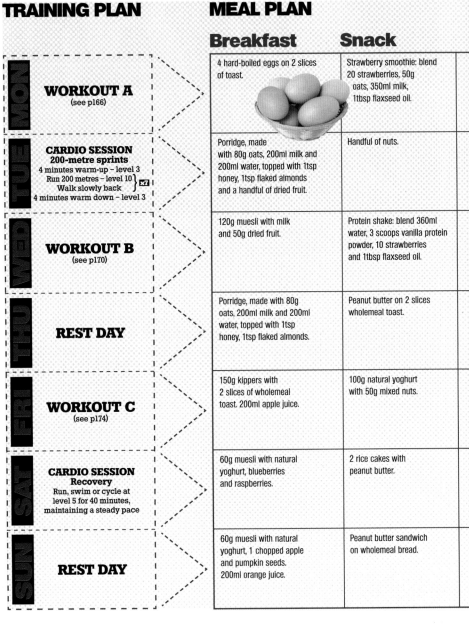

MON

WORKOUT A
(see p166)

TUE

CARDIO SESSION
200-metre sprints
4 minutes warm-up – level 3
Run 200 metres – level 10 }×7
Walk slowly back
4 minutes warm down – level 3

WED

WORKOUT B
(see p170)

THU

REST DAY

FRI

WORKOUT C
(see p174)

SAT

CARDIO SESSION
Recovery
Run, swim or cycle at level 5 for 40 minutes, maintaining a steady pace

SUN

REST DAY

MEAL PLAN

Breakfast	Snack
4 hard-boiled eggs on 2 slices of toast.	Strawberry smoothie: blend 20 strawberries, 50g oats, 350ml milk, 1tbsp flaxseed oil.
Porridge, made with 80g oats, 200ml milk and 200ml water, topped with 1tsp honey, 1tsp flaked almonds and a handful of dried fruit.	Handful of nuts.
120g muesli with milk and 50g dried fruit.	Protein shake: blend 360ml water, 3 scoops vanilla protein powder, 10 strawberries and 1tbsp flaxseed oil.
Porridge, made with 80g oats, 200ml milk and 200ml water, topped with 1tsp honey, 1tsp flaked almonds.	Peanut butter on 2 slices wholemeal toast.
150g kippers with 2 slices of wholemeal toast. 200ml apple juice.	100g natural yoghurt with 50g mixed nuts.
60g muesli with natural yoghurt, blueberries and raspberries.	2 rice cakes with peanut butter.
60g muesli with natural yoghurt, 1 chopped apple and pumpkin seeds. 200ml orange juice.	Peanut butter sandwich on wholemeal bread.

WEEK 4 | WEEK 5 | WEEK 6 | WEEK 7 | WEEK 8 | WEEK 9 | WEEK 10 | WEEK 11 | WEEK 12

Lunch	Snack	Dinner	Snack	Total
Salmon, cucumber and mayonnaise sandwich.	Protein shake: blend 360ml water, 3 scoops vanilla protein powder, 10 strawberries and 1tbsp flaxseed oil.	Chicken curry made with 200g chicken. 85g brown rice.	1 pear and a handful of seeds.	**3,320 calories** 197g protein 253g carbs 99g fat
Turkey and cheese baguette. 1 pot of natural yoghurt.	125g hummus with 10g carrots, 20g celery and 25g peppers.	Spaghetti bolognese, made with 200g minced beef. 75g dried spaghetti. Green side salad.	200ml of milk.	**3,212 calories** 199g protein 430g carbs 115g fat
Chicken and mushroom pasta.	Apple and 10 almonds.	300g lean roast beef, 300g potatoes, 100g veg	Pot of natural yogurt	**3,569 calories** 245g protein 385g carbs 94g fat
Steak and cheese wholemeal baguette.	3 celery sticks, 2 carrots and 50g hummus.	2 jacket potatoes with cottage cheese and tuna. Side salad.	200ml of milk.	**3,015 calories,** 117g protein, 332g carbs, 138g fat
Spanish omelette using 4 eggs, potatoes, peppers and onions. Side salad.	1 chopped banana and 25g pumpkin seeds.	2 Cajun chicken breasts with 85g brown rice and vegetables. 40g 70% cocoa dark organic chocolate.	Protein shake made with 200ml semi-skimmed milk.	**2,975 calories,** 130g protein 291g carbs 114g fat
Steak and cheese wholemeal baguette.	50g beef jerky. 1 apple.	½ pepperoni pizza with salad. 2 pancakes with vanilla ice cream.	50g mixed nuts and seeds.	**2,912 calories** 156g protein 349g carbs 103g fat
Grilled chicken with couscous, peppers, courgettes, carrots, onions, pine nuts and apricots.	Nectarine smoothie: blend 50ml apple juice, 1 nectarine, ½ punnet of raspberries, 1tsp honey and 100ml natural yoghurt. Cereal bar.	Roast beef with 5 roast potatoes, carrots, broccoli, cauliflower, peas and parsnips.	200ml vanilla ice cream.	**2,989 calories** 149g protein 297g carbs 117g fat

WORKOUT A

This workout will hit muscle groups right across your body. Watch out for the cluster sets on the deadlift: each cluster is five mini-sets of four reps with only ten seconds rest between each. Use a weight that you would normally pick to do three sets of tens reps.

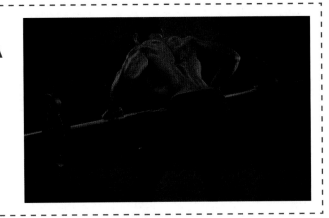

Warm-up Ten minutes of gentle cardio followed by dynamic stretches (see p13)

Exercise	Sets	Reps	Tempo	Rest	Weight
1 Cluster deadlift	**3** clusters	**4**	**311**	**60** secs	
2 Lunge to press	**3**	**5** each leg	**211**	**60** secs	
3 Pull-up	**3**	**6-10**	**311**	**60** secs	**n/a**
4 Reverse grip triceps extension	**3**	**8-10**	**311**	**60** secs	
5 Weighted crunch	**3**	**8-10**	**311**	**60** secs	
6 Gym ball press-up	**3**	**10-12**	**311**	**60** secs	**n/a**

Warm down and stretch Ten minutes of gentle cardio plus static stretches (20 seconds each). Focus on quads, hams, glutes, traps, lats, shoulders, triceps, abs (see p14)

Notes

① **Cluster deadlift**

Target: quads, glutes, hamstrings, back, core

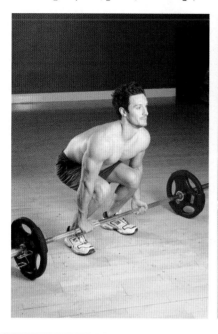 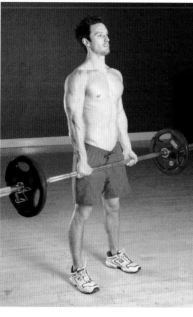

- Start with your feet shoulder width apart, grasp the bar outside your knees with an overhand or alternate grip.
- Position the bar close to your shins with your shoulders directly over it and keep looking forward.
- Ensure you keep your back flat, your shoulders retracted and your core braced.
- Start the lift by pushing with your glutes and pushing down through the heels.
- Keeping your shoulders back, the bar should rise up your shins, as it passes your knees, push your hips forward.

② **Lunge to press**

Target: quads, glutes, hamstrings, shoulders, triceps

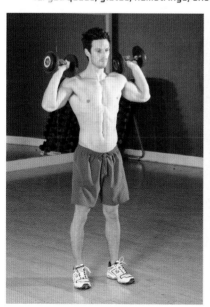 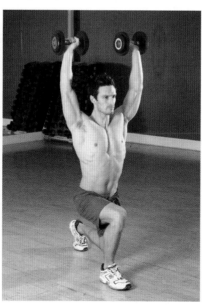

- Stand upright with your feet apart and your toes facing forward, keep your core braced throughout.
- Hold the dumb-bells at shoulder level with your palms facing forward.
- Take a big step forward, making sure your front knee is over your front foot, sink down until your back knee almost touches the floor.
- Maintaining a natural arch in your spine, press the weights directly overhead.
- Push off your front foot to return to the start while lowering the weights.

❸ Pull-up

Target: lats, traps, rhomboids

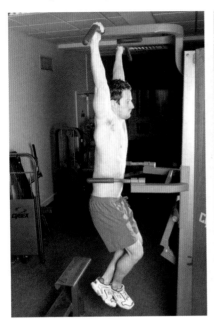 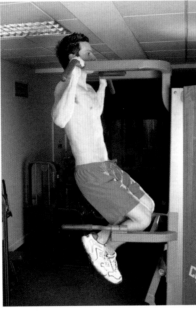

● Grip the bar with an overhand grip just wider than shoulder width apart.

● Extend your arms fully, letting your body hang straight down without swinging.

● Pull up until your chin is over the bar, squeezing your lats as you rise.

● Lower slowly without swinging.

❹ Reverse grip triceps extension

Target: triceps

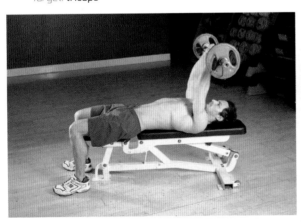 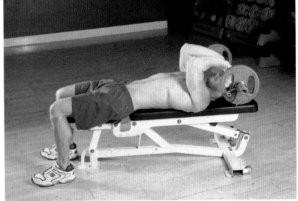

● Lie on a bench with your core braced, knees bent at 90° and feet flat on the ground.

● Hold the EZ-bar over your head, not your chest, with an underhand grip, wrists turned in slightly.

● Without arching your back, lower the bar slowly behind your head while keeping your upper arms vertical.

● Reverse the motion to press the bar back up, squeezing your triceps at the top of the move.

⑤ Weighted crunch

Target: **upper abdominals**

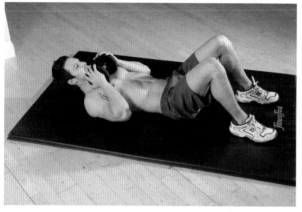 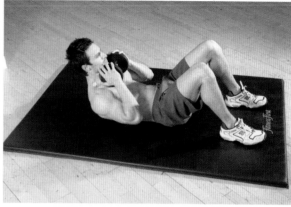

● Lie with your feet flat on the floor, knees bent at 90° and head off the mat.

● Hold a dumb-bell or weight plate to your chest.

● Keeping your lower back in contact with the mat, contract your abs to lift your shoulders off the mat, curling your chest towards your knees.

● Pause at the top of the move, squeeze your abs and lower slowly to the start.

⑥ Gym ball press-up

Target: **pecs, triceps**

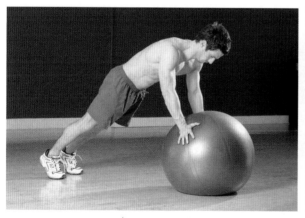 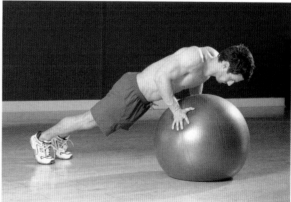

● Brace your core to keep your body in a straight line from head to heels.

● Grip the sides of the ball with your hands roughly in line with your shoulders.

● Slowly lower your body towards the ball, controlling any wobbling, then press up powerfully.

WORKOUT B

In this workout you'll use a Smith machine to perform your bench press clusters. This will help you to stick to your ten-second rest periods without having to rack and unrack a barbell, as you would with a standard bench press. For each cluster do four reps, rest for ten seconds and repeat five times.

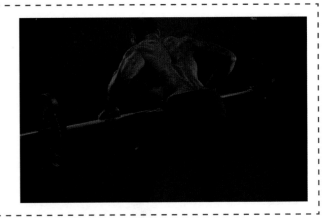

Warm-up Ten minutes of gentle cardio followed by dynamic stretches (see p13)

Exercise		Sets	Reps	Tempo	Rest	Weight
1 Cluster Smith machine press		**3** clusters	**4**	**311**	**60** secs	
2 Cable woodchop		**3**	**10** each side	**311**	**60** secs	
3 High pull		**3**	**8-10**	**31X**	**60** secs	
4 Split squat		**3**	**6** each leg	**311**	**60** secs	
5 Barbell rollout		**3**	**8-10**	**311**	**60** secs	**n/a**
6 Barbell curl		**3**	**8-10**	**311**	**60** secs	

Warm down and stretch Ten minutes of gentle cardio plus static stretches (20 seconds each). Focus on chest, quads, hams, glutes, traps, biceps, abs (see p14)

Notes

❶ Cluster Smith machine press

Target: **pecs, triceps**

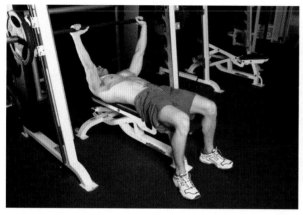 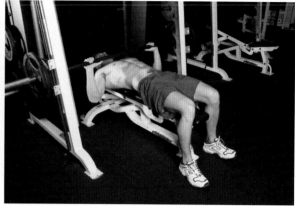

● Position the bench so the bar is directly over your chest.

● Lie with your knees bent at 90°, your feet flat on the floor and your core braced.

● Grip the bar wider than shoulder width, retract your shoulder blades

and lower the bar to your chest slowly then press up powerfully.

● Maintain a natural arch in your back throughout. There should be just enough room to slip a few fingers between your lower back and the bench.

❷ Cable woodchop

Target: **abdominals, core**

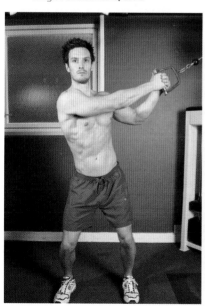 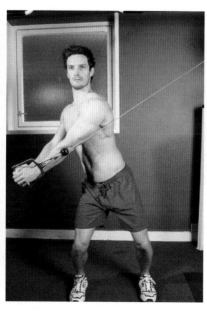

● Stand side-on to a high cable, turn your torso towards it and grip the handle with both hands.

● Keeping your arms as straight as possible, use your core muscles to draw the cable down and across your body.

● Reverse the motion under control to the start.

❸ High pull

Target: **hamstrings, glutes, calves, back, shoulders**

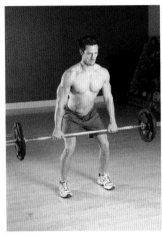
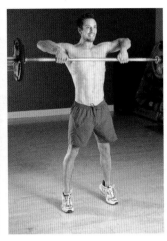

● Stand with your feet shoulder width apart, your back straight, shoulders back and core braced.

● Grip the bar just outside your knees, lean forward from the hips, not the waist, and bend your knees to initiate the move.

● Pull the bar up in front of you powerfully, rising up onto your toes to gain more power and keeping your elbows high.

● Lower the bar in a controlled manner and return to the start.

❹ Split squat

Target: **quads, hamstrings, glutes**

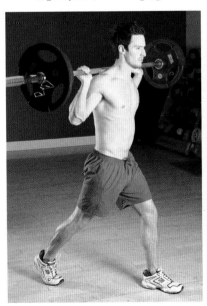
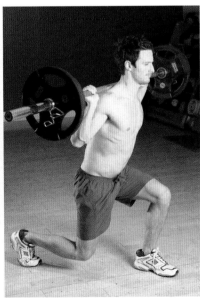

● Start in a split stance with both feet facing forward, back upright and core braced.

● Rest the bar on the back of your shoulders and keep your elbows back to retract your shoulder blades.

● Sink down until your back knee almost touches the floor and your front knee bends to 90°.

⑤ **Barbell rollout**

Target: **core, lower back**

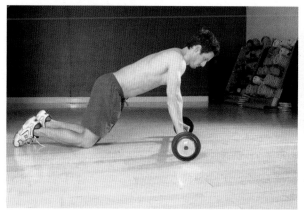 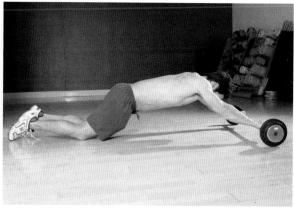

● Start with the barbell directly beneath your shoulders, gripping it just wider than shoulder width apart.

● Keeping your back and your arms straight throughout, roll the bar as far out as you can before you feel you might break

form, then reverse the move.

● Use your abdominals to control the movement, making it slow and deliberate.

⑥ **Barbell curl**

Target: **biceps**

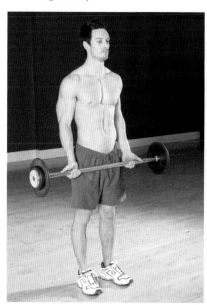 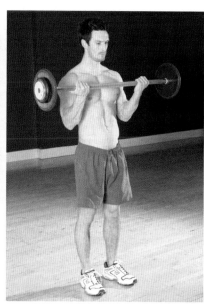

● Stand tall with your shoulders back and your core muscles braced for support.

● Grip the bar just outside your hips and keep your elbows tucked into your sides with a slight bend in them.

● Lift the bar without rocking back and forth for momentum, stop before your forearms are vertical and lower slowly.

WORKOUT C

As in the previous workout you'll use the Smith machine to manage your cluster sets, only this time you'll be doing squats instead of bench presses. Pick a weight that you would normally use to do three sets of ten, then do five sets of four with just ten seconds' rest in between. That's one cluster.

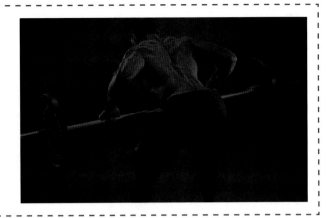

Warm-up Ten minutes of gentle cardio followed by dynamic stretches (see p13)

Exercise		Sets	Reps	Tempo	Rest	Weight
① Cluster Smith squat		3 clusters	4	311	60 secs	
② Romanian deadlift to row		3	8-10	311	60 secs	
③ Arnold press		3	8-10	311	60 secs	
④ Incline dumb-bell flye		3	8-10	311	60 secs	
⑤ Close grip lat pull down to triceps press down		3	8-10	311	60 secs	
⑥ Raised side plank		2	6 each side	212	60 secs	n/a

Warm down and stretch Ten minutes of gentle cardio plus static stretches (20 seconds each). Focus on quads, hams, glutes, traps, chest, shoulders, triceps, lower back (see p14)

Notes

❶ Cluster Smith squat

Target: quads, glutes

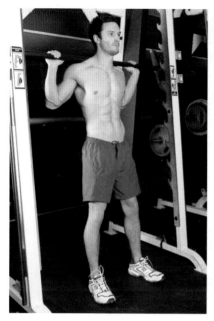
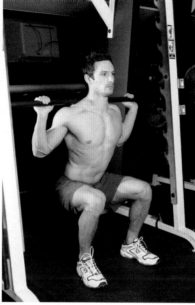

● Place your feet shoulder width apart and slightly in front of your body to put more emphasis on your quads.

● Rest the bar on the back of your shoulders, not your neck, and keep your elbows back.

● Look forward, brace your core and unlock the bar from the rack.

● Maintaining a natural arch in your back, lower until your thighs are parallel to the floor.

● Push back up through your heels.

❷ Romanian deadlift to row

Target: hamstrings, glutes, core, back, arms

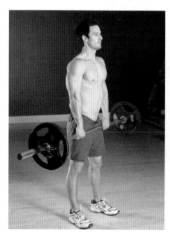
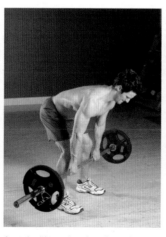
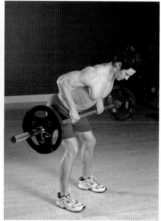

● Stand with your feet shoulder width apart, keep looking forward, with your shoulders back and core braced.

● Grip the bar just outside your hips and initiate the move by leaning forward

from the hips rather than the waist.

● Allow a slight bend in your knees, keep your back straight and push your hips back as the bar travels down your shins.

● Keep your torso still and pull the bar up to your abdomen, squeezing your shoulder blades together at the top.

③ Arnold press

Target: **deltoids**

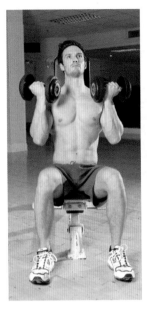
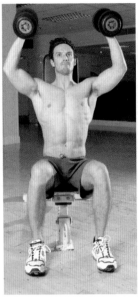
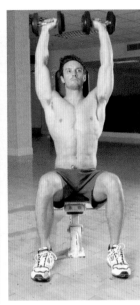

● Sit on a bench with your lower back and shoulders pressed against the pad, keep your feet flat on the floor.

● Hold the dumb-bells at shoulder height, palms facing in and elbows to the front.

● As you press the weights directly overhead rotate your palms so that they finish facing forward.

● Reverse the motion back to the start.

④ Incline dumb-bell flye

Target: **pecs**

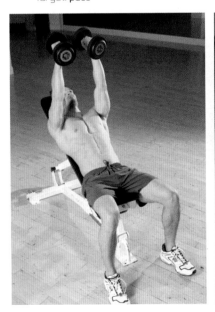
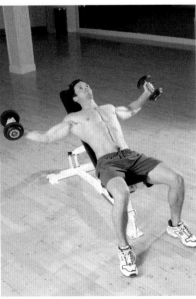

● Lie on a bench set at 30-45° with your feet flat on the floor.

● Hold the dumb-bells directly over your chest with your palms facing each other, keeping a slight bend in your elbows.

● Without arching your back, lower the dumb-bells in an arc out to the sides as far as is comfortable.

● Use your pectoral muscles to reverse the movement back to the start.

⑤ Close grip lat pull down to triceps press down

Target: **lats, traps, rhomboids, triceps**

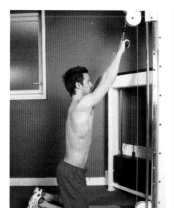
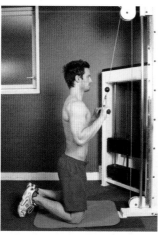
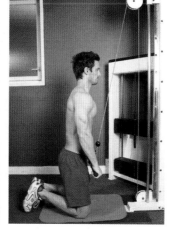

- Grip a short bar with your palms facing away from you.
- Keeping your body upright, retract your shoulder blades and pull your elbows into your sides.
- Press the bar down without moving your elbows or upper arms.
- Reverse the motion in a controlled manner.

⑥ Raised side plank

Target: **core, obliques**

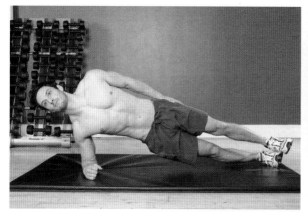
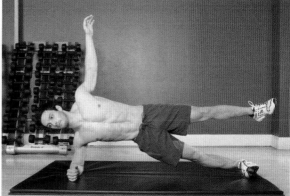

- With your elbow positioned directly below your shoulder, hold your body in a straight line from head to heels.
- Lift your free arm and leg but don't let the arm go beyond vertical.
- Hold this position for a count of two before lowering slowly.

WEEK 12
JUMP TO IT

You've made it to the final week! Congratulations. To finish off, we'll be introducing plyometrics to your workouts. These are exercises that require you to place the muscle under tension before performing the concentric part of the move explosively, such as jumping off the floor. This hits your fast-twitch muscle fibres – the ones with the most potential for growth. It will also get your heart pumping, to stoke your fat-burning furnaces. By the time you finish this week, you should be feeling stronger, faster and fitter – with a body that you are proud to show off.

TRAINING PLAN

MON

WORKOUT A
(see p180)

TUE

CARDIO SESSION
24-minute running intervals
4 minutes warm-up – level 3
2 minutes fast – level 7
2 minutes slow – level 4 } x3
4 minutes warm down – level 3

WED

WORKOUT B
(see p184)

THU

REST DAY

FRI

WORKOUT C
(see p188)

SAT

CARDIO SESSION
Recovery
Run, swim or cycle at level 5 for 40 minutes, maintaining a steady pace

SUN

WELL-EARNED REST DAY

MEAL PLAN

Breakfast	Snack
4 scrambled eggs with 100g smoked salmon. 2 slices wholemeal toast.	1 small pot of natural yoghurt. 300g almonds and mixed dried fruit.
120g muesli with 50g dried fruit. 250ml milk.	1 slice bread with peanut butter. 1 apple.
120g muesli with 50g dried fruit. 250ml milk.	Protein shake: blend 360ml water, 3 scoops vanilla protein powder, 10 strawberries and 1tbsp flaxseed oil.
4 hard-boiled eggs on 2 slices toast. Handful of dried fruit.	Strawberry smoothie: blend 20 strawberries, 50g oats, 350ml milk, 1tbsp flaxseed oil.
3 poached eggs on 2 slices wholemeal toast.	55g beef jerky. 1 apple.
Porridge, made with 80g oats, 200ml milk and 200ml water, topped with 1tsp honey, 1tsp flaked almonds.	Peanut butter on wholemeal toast.
50g muesli with apricots and semi-skimmed milk.	1 cereal bar. 1 orange.

Lunch	Snack	Dinner	Snack	Total
1 jacket potato with 200g tuna and ½ tin of sweetcorn. 1 banana.	1 slices of toast with peanut butter.	300g chicken, 200g rice and stir-fried vegetables.	1 slice of bread with peanut butter.	**3,337 calories,** 131g protein, 163g carbs, 49g fat
Spanish omelette made with 5 egg whites, ½ potato, ½ red pepper, ½ onion and ½ tomato.	1 slice of bread with peanut butter.	½ meat pizza with avocado and feta salad (½ avocado, 75g feta and 1 tomato) dressed with 1tbsp balsamic vinegar.	1 protein bar.	**3,380 calories** 118g protein 268g carbs 110g fat
Chicken and mushroom pasta.	1 small pot of natural yoghurt.	300g lean roast beef, 300g potatoes, 100g mixed vegetables.	10 almonds.	**3,569 calories,** 245g protein, 385g carbs, 94g fat
Salmon, cucumber and mayonnaise sandwich.	Protein shake: blend 360ml water, 3 scoops vanilla protein powder, 10 strawberries and 1tbsp flaxseed oil.	Chicken bhuna curry with 85g brown rice.	1 pear.	**3,320 calories,** 197g protein, 253g carbs, 99g fat
120g smoked salmon with spinach, cucumber, and mixed salad leaves. 2 wholemeal pitta breads.	75g natural organic yoghurt with 25g muesli, 60g strawberries and 20g hazelnuts.	Beef tacos (200g lean minced beef, ½ packet of taco spice mix, 1tbsp low-fat cheddar and 1tbsp salsa). Serve with a green salad.	Coconut smoothie: blend 100ml coconut milk, 50ml orange juice, ½ pineapple, 1 banana, 75ml semi-skimmed milk and 1tbsp oats.	**2,953 calories** 191g protein 255g carbs 136g fat
Steak and cheese wholemeal baguette.	3 celery sticks, 2 carrots and 50g hummus. 200ml milk.	2 jacket potatoes with cottage cheese and tuna. Side salad.	Peanut butter on wholemeal toast.	**3,015 calories,** 117g protein, 332g carbs, 138g fat
2 jacket potatoes with tuna and mayonnaise. 250ml cranberry juice.	Peanut butter on 2 slices of wholemeal toast.	Turkey stir-fry with peppers, mushrooms, onions and courgettes. 1 pint of lager.	1 cereal bar.	**2,950 calories** 111g protein 324g carbs 67g fat

WORKOUT A

Aim to perform these exercises with fast, dynamic moves. However, be sure not to compromise good form for speed. You'll need to keep your core muscles tight to stabilise your body during the exercises.

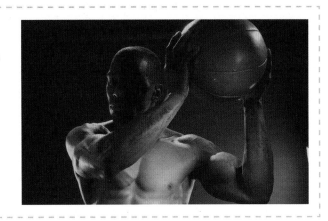

Warm-up Ten minutes of gentle cardio followed by dynamic stretches (see p13)

Exercise		Sets	Reps	Tempo	Rest	Weight
① Clap press-up		3	6-8	21X	60 secs	n/a
② Step up and jump		3	6-8 each leg	21X	60 secs	n/a
③ Medicine ball throw downs		3	8 each side	21X	60 secs	
④ Hang clean		3	8-10	31X	60 secs	
⑤ Split squat to one-arm row		3	10 each side	311	60 secs	
⑥ Shoulder press with rotation		3	5 each side	311	60 secs	

Warm down and stretch Ten minutes of gentle cardio plus static stretches (20 seconds each). Focus on chest, triceps, quads, hams, glutes, traps, shoulders, abs, lower back (see p14)

Notes

① Clap press-up

Target: pecs, triceps

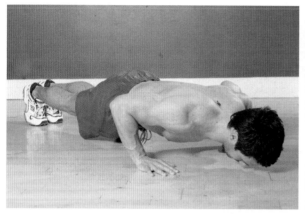
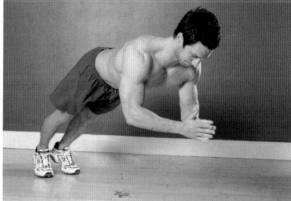

● Position your hands just wider than shoulder width apart and keep your body straight.

● Lower into a press-up, ensuring your elbows stay back.

● Push up so you leave the floor, clap, and go straight into the next rep.

② Step up and jump

Target: glutes, quads, hamstrings

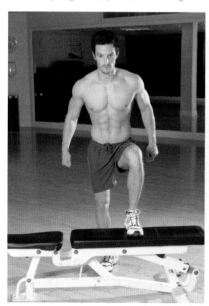
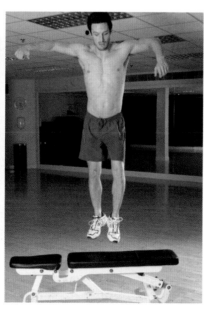

● Using a bench no higher than knee height, keep your back upright and look forward.

● Place one foot on the bench and push off it powerfully to jump into the air.

● Land safely on the floor and re-set before repeating.

③ Medicine ball throw downs

Target: obliques

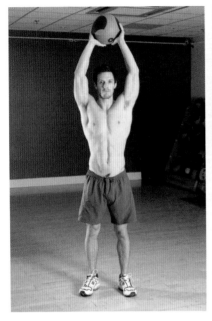 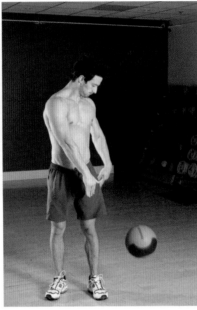

● Stand with the ball held over your head, back straight and core engaged.

● Throw the ball down hard to the side, catch it on the bounce and repeat to the other side.

④ Hang clean

Target: hamstrings, glutes, calves, back, shoulders

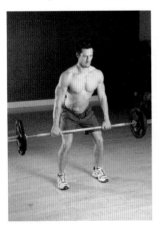 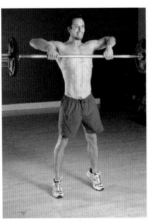 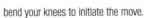 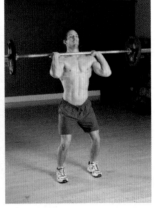

● Stand with your feet shoulder width apart, your back straight, shoulders back and core braced.

● Grip the bar just outside your knees, lean forward from the hips, not the waist, and

bend your knees to initiate the move.

● Pull the bar up in front of you powerfully, rising up onto your toes to gain more power and keeping your elbows high.

● Bend your knees to duck under the bar at

its highest point, flipping it onto your fingers and catching it on top of your chest.

● Stand up straight and reset the bar before repeating.

⑤ Split squat to one-arm row

Target: legs, back, arms, shoulders, core

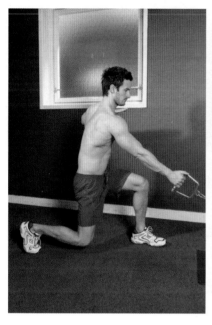
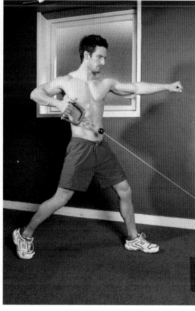

● Start in a lunge position with your left leg forward and your right hand gripping a low cable handle.

● Turn your body towards the cable, keep your head upright and your core braced.

● Without moving your feet, stand up, draw the cable back to your side and retract your shoulder blade while turning your body away from the cable.

⑥ Shoulder press with rotation

Target: deltoids, core

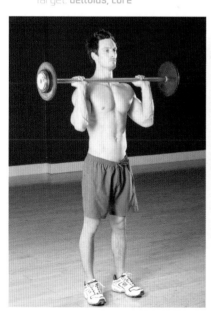
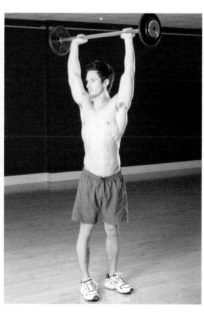

● Stand with your feet shoulder width apart, your body upright, core braced and head looking straight ahead.

● Grip the bar just wider than shoulder width apart and hold it on your upper chest.

● As you press the bar directly overhead rotate your body to the side, using your core muscles to control the motion.

● Slowly return to the start, alternate sides with each rep.

WORKOUT B

Only two more workouts to go! As with the previous workout, these exercises should be performed explosively while maintaining good form. It's worth practising the moves with light weights (or no weights) before starting your sets, just to get your body prepared for the work to come.

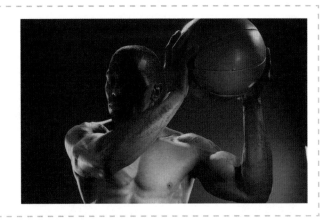

Warm-up Ten minutes of gentle cardio followed by dynamic stretches (see p13)

Exercise		Sets	Reps	Tempo	Rest	Weight
1 Jump squat		3	8-10	21X	60 secs	
2 Ballistic bench press		3	8-10	31X	60 secs	
3 One-arm dumb-bell snatch		3	6-8 each arm	31X	60 secs	
4 Bent-over flye		3	8-10	311	60 secs	
5 Jackknife		3	8-10	31X	60 secs	n/a
6 Cable split squat to overhead press		3	8 each side	311	60 secs	

Warm down and stretch Ten minutes of gentle cardio plus static stretches (20 seconds each). Focus on quads, hams, glutes, chest, triceps, traps, shoulders, abs, lower back (see p14)

Notes

① Jump squat

Target: quads, glutes, hamstrings

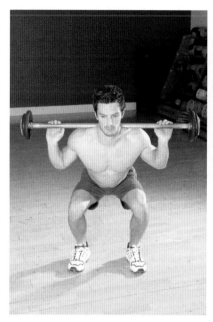
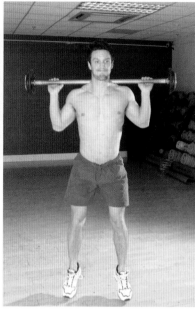

- Stand with your feet shoulder width apart, your toes turned out slightly and your core braced.
- Rest a light barbell on the back of your shoulders, not your neck, gripping it close to your shoulders.
- Maintain a natural arch in your back, keep your elbows retracted and look forward throughout the movement.
- Lower until your thighs are parallel to the floor, keeping your knees in line with your feet, then push back up explosively to jump off the ground.

② Ballistic bench press

Target: pecs, triceps

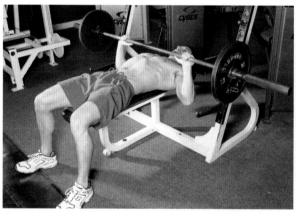

- Lie on the bench with your knees bent at 90°, your feet flat on the floor and your core braced.
- Grip the bar wider than shoulder width,

with your shoulder blades retracted.
- Maintain a natural arch in your back, there should just be enough room to slip a few fingers between

your lower back and the bench.
- Lower the bar to your chest slowly then press it up quickly but under control.

③ One-arm dumb-bell snatch

Target: hamstrings, glutes, calves, back, shoulders, arms

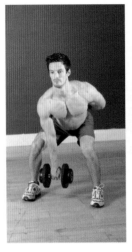 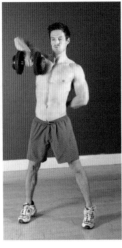 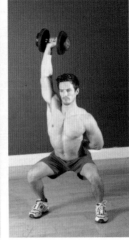 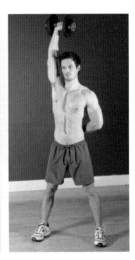

● Start in a deadlift position, holding one dumb-bell between your legs.

● Ensure you keep your back flat, your core braced and your shoulders square.

● Lift the weight in front of you powerfully, rising up onto your toes to gain more power and keeping your elbow high.

● Squat beneath the weight at its highest point to catch it with a straight arm then stand up straight.

④ Bent-over flye

Target: traps, lats, rhomboids

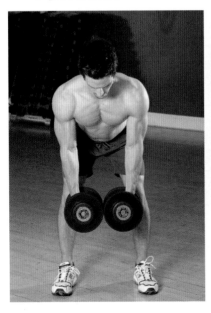 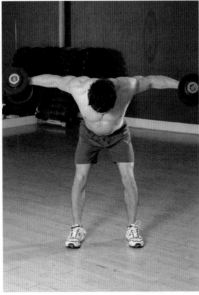

● Start with your core braced, your back straight and your shoulder blades retracted.

● With your knees slightly bent, lean forward from the hips, rather than the waist, keep your back straight.

● Keeping a slight bend in your elbows, raise the weights straight out to the sides without moving your upper body.

● Squeeze your shoulder blades at the top of the movement and lower slowly.

⑤ Jackknife

Target: abdominals

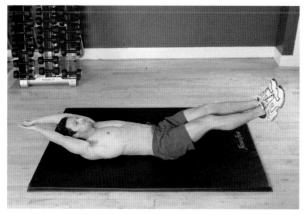 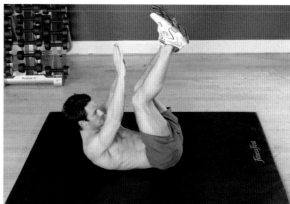

● Start with your arms behind your head, held off the floor, and your feet together, also off the floor.

● Contract your abs to bring your arms and legs up to meet above your stomach, keep your legs as straight as you can.

● Squeeze your abs hard at the top of the move and slowly lower to the start.

⑥ Cable split squat to overhead press

Target: quads, glutes, hamstrings, core, pecs, shoulders

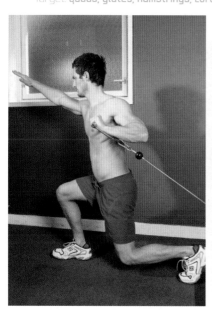 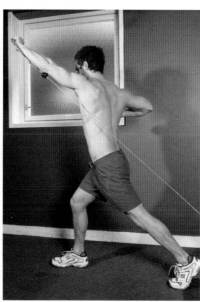

● Start in a lunge position, facing away from a low cable, with your right leg forward and your left hand gripping the handle.

● Twist your torso towards the cable, keep your head upright and your core braced.

● Without moving your feet, stand up, pressing the handle upwards at 45° while turning your body away from the cable.

WORKOUT C

This is it! The last workout. Make it a good one. Once again you should perform the exercises with fast, dynamic movements while still ensuring that you maintain good form at all times.

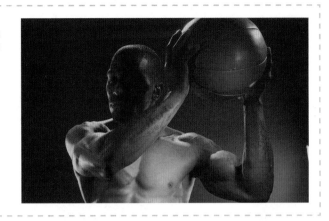

Warm-up Ten minutes of gentle cardio followed by dynamic stretches (see p13)

Exercise		Sets	Reps	Tempo	Rest	Weight
① Medicine ball sledgehammer		3	10-12	X0X	60 secs	
② T press-up		3	6 each side	21X	60 secs	
③ Jumping lunge		3	6 each side	21X	60 secs	n/a
④ Inverted row		3	10-12	311	60 secs	n/a
⑤ Woodchop lunge		3	8 each side	21X	60 secs	
⑥ Bicycles		3	40 secs	101	60 secs	n/a

Warm down and stretch Ten minutes of gentle cardio plus static stretches (20 seconds each). Focus on quads, hams, glutes, chest, triceps, lats, biceps, shoulders, abs, lower back (see p14)

Notes

① Medicine ball sledgehammer
Target: whole body

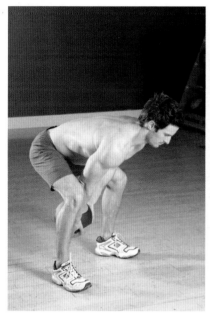
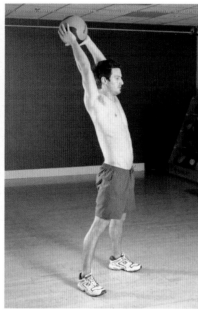

● Stand straight with a medicine ball held above your head and brace your core.

● Bring the ball down powerfully through your legs, bending at the knees and hips and keeping your back flat.

● Reverse the motion and return to the start.

② T press-up
Target: chest, shoulders, arms, core

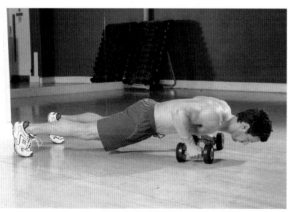
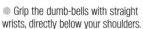
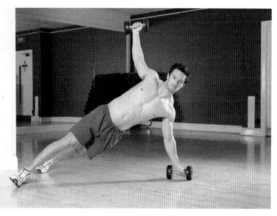

● Grip the dumb-bells with straight wrists, directly below your shoulders.

● Position your feet shoulder width apart and don't let your hips sag.

● Keep your body in a straight line and your elbows tucked into your sides.

● Push up powerfully and twist your body, rolling onto the sides of your feet while keeping your body straight.

● Raise the dumb-bell overhead with a straight arm, return to the start and repeat on the other side.

③ Jumping lunge

Target: quads, glutes, hamstrings

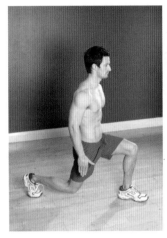 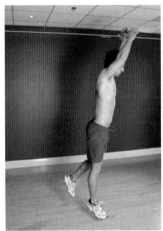

● Start in a lunge position, feet facing forward, back knee almost touching the floor and your front knee over your front foot.

● Jump up, raise your hands to gain height, and swap leg positions in mid air.

● Land in another lunge and go straight into the next jump.

④ Inverted row

Target: mid traps, lats, rhomboids

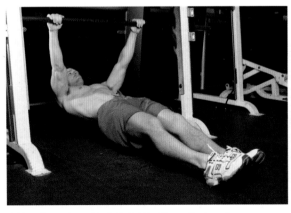 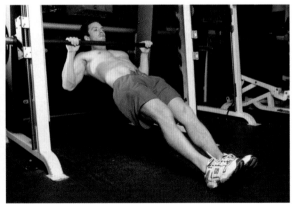

● Hang from a bar set to thigh height with your heels resting on the ground and your body straight from head to heels.

● Pull your chest up to the bar and squeeze your shoulder blades together, return slowly to the start position.

⑤ **Woodchop lunge**

Target: abdominals, lower back, core, quads, glutes, hamstrings, shoulders

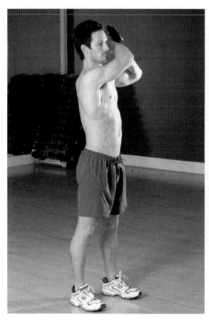 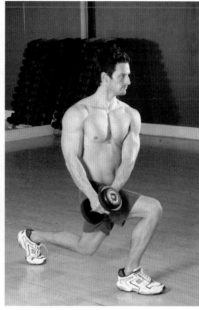

● Stand up straight holding a dumb-bell in both hands over one shoulder.

● Step forward into a lunge and chop the weight down and across your body.

● Be careful to keep your back straight, your feet pointing forwards and your front knee over your front foot.

⑥ **Bicycles**

Target: abdominals

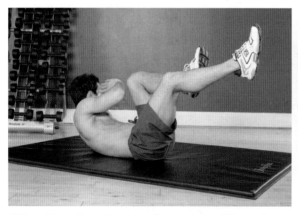 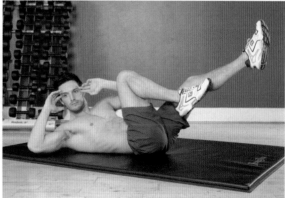

● Start with your fingers by your temples, crunch up to bring your right elbow to your left knee while extending your right leg.

● Twist your torso to the other side as you crunch your left elbow to your right knee and extend your left leg.

● Perform this movement in a quick but controlled manner, being careful not to strain your neck.

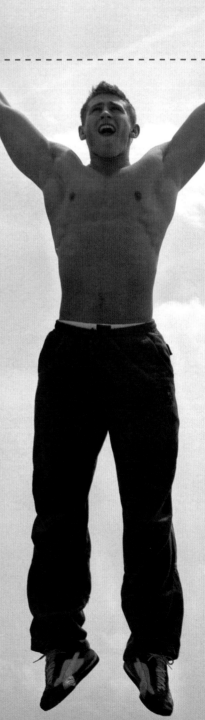

Congratulations!

You've made it to the end of the Body Challenge...

After 12 weeks of hard training and good eating you should be looking and feeling better than ever before. So where do you go from here? To maintain the body you've built, you'll need to continue to exercise regularly and watch what you eat. That doesn't mean that you can't treat yourself – we all need a blow-out now and then – but try to keep these tips in mind to keep your body in great shape.

★ Make treats for treat-time only
A tub of ice cream or a double pepperoni pizza isn't going to derail all your good work – if you have them occasionally. Aim to make most of your meals unprocessed, high in protein, low in saturated fat and with a good range of fruit and veg.

★ Limit your booze intake
They don't call it a beer belly for nothing. Alcohol is the quickest way to pile on the pounds, so don't celebrate a good session at the gym with a visit to the pub.

★ Make exercise regular
It's better to do three short sessions a week than one monster workout. Find a way to fit exercise around your daily schedule, then it won't feel like it's eating into valuable social or family time.

★ Keep mixing it up
This programme has given you a wide selection of exercises for all body parts. Use these and others (look out for more in *Men's Fitness* magazine every month) to create your own workouts and challenge your muscles in new ways.

★ Keep upping the ante
Every four or five weeks aim to lift 5-10 per cent more weight than you have been, or increase the intensity of your cardio sessions. This will keep your body adapting to new stresses, making you fitter and stronger all the time.

★ Have fun
The exercise regime you stick with is the one you enjoy. Listen to music, rope in your friends, enter a race or competition – anything that helps you to see your training as fun rather than a chore.

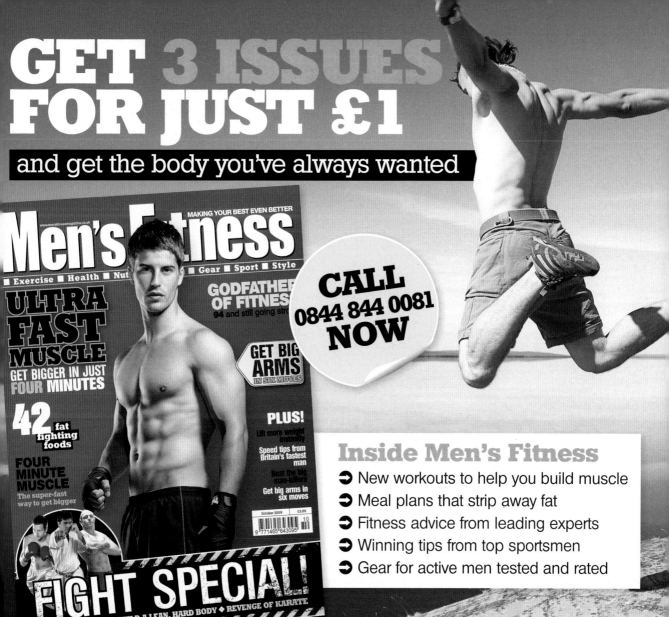

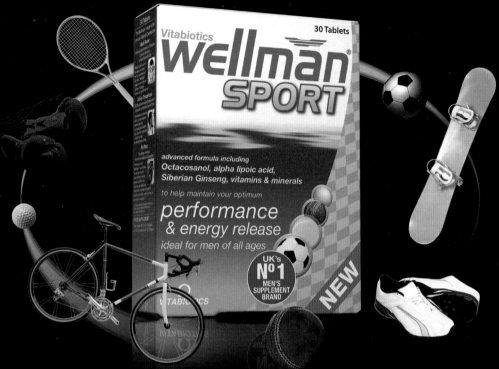

the best sportsmen

NEW

Vitabiotics

wellman®
SPORT

30 Tablets

advanced formula including
Octacosanol, alpha lipoic acid,
Siberian Ginseng, vitamins & minerals

to help maintain your optimum

performance
& energy release

ideal for men of all ages

UK's
№1
MEN'S
SUPPLEMENT
BRAND

NEW

use the best equipment

Wellman® Sport is designed to help support the most important piece of sporting equipment there is – you. Its comprehensive formula safeguards your nutritional requirement to help sustain the body whilst training. The advanced one-a-day tablet replaces your usual multivitamin and includes natural plant isolate Octacosanol, Alpha Lipoic Acid for advanced antioxidant protection and B-complex vitamins to help support energy release. For further information, visit Wellman.co.uk.

Wellman® Sport is new from Wellman®, the UK's leading supplement range for men.

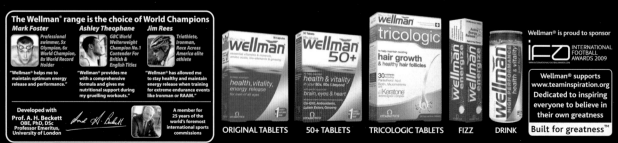

The Wellman® range is the choice of World Champions

Mark Foster
Professional swimmer, 5x Olympian, 6x World Champion, 8x World Record Holder

"Wellman® helps me to maintain optimum energy release and performance."

Developed with
Prof. A. H. Beckett
OBE, PhD, DSc
Professor Emeritus,
University of London

Ashley Theophane
GBC World Welterweight Champion No.1 Contender For British & English Titles

"Wellman® provides me with a comprehensive formula and gives me nutritional support during my gruelling workouts."

Jim Rees
Triathlete, Ironman, Race Across America elite athlete

"Wellman® has allowed me to stay healthy and maintain energy release when training for extreme endurance events like Ironman or RAAM."

A member for 25 years of the world's foremost international sports commissions

ORIGINAL TABLETS — wellman® essential vitamins & minerals, amino acids, bio-elements & ginseng — health, vitality, energy release for men of all ages

50+ TABLETS — wellman® 50+ health & vitality in your 50s, 60s & beyond, brain, eyes & heart — Co-Q10, Antioxidants, Lutein Esters, Ginseng

TRICOLOGIC TABLETS — wellman® tricologic — hair growth & healthy hair follicles — Keratone®

FIZZ — wellman® energize

DRINK — wellman®

Wellman® is proud to sponsor

iFZ INTERNATIONAL FOOTBALL AWARDS 2009

Wellman® supports
www.teaminspiration.org
Dedicated to inspiring everyone to believe in their own greatness

Built for greatness™

www.wellman.co.uk

The Wellman® range is available from selected Boots, Superdrug, supermarkets, Holland & Barrett, GNC, Lloydspharmacy, pharmacies & health stores.
Vitamin supplements may benefit those with nutritionally inadequate diets.

Britain's leading supplements for specific life stages

THE QUEEN'S AWARDS FOR ENTERPRISE 2009

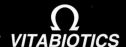

Ω
VITABIOTICS